Contents

**Section 3    History-related topics (topics based on key points in history)**                                   **73**

    Chapter 14:  The Department of Health, and events up to the early 1990s    75

    Chapter 15:  The NHS Plan: precursors and consequences, including standards    85

    Chapter 16:  Other bodies and philosophies which evolved from the NHS Plan    99

**Section 4    Important concepts and relevant bodies**                                   **119**

    Chapter 17:  Revalidation, appraisal, job planning and performance management    121

    Chapter 18:  Other important bodies and concepts    133

**Section 5    Miscellaneous hot topics**                                   **143**

    Chapter 19:  Medical education    145

    Chapter 20:  Principles of leadership and management for doctors    149

    Chapter 21:  The Trust management structure    157

    Chapter 22:  Financial issues    163

    Chapter 23:  Additional qualities required of a Consultant    167

    Chapter 24:  Clinical governance and quality    179

    Chapter 25:  Continuing education and development    199

    Chapter 26:  Legal and ethical issues    203

    Chapter 27:  Other key reports    215

**Section 6    Ending the interview**                                   **231**

**Appendix    References**                                   **233**

    Useful websites    237

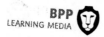

www.bma.org.uk/library

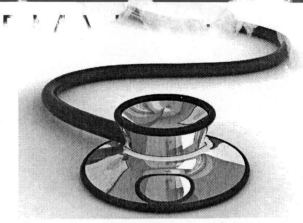

# Succeeding in your Consultant Medical Interview

A comprehensive guide to interview question topics and NHS issues

## Second Edition

**Robert Ghosh**

D1333846

**BPP**
LEARNING MEDIA

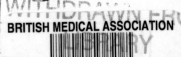

**First edition 2009**
**Second edition December 2011**

ISBN 9781 4453 8228 9
Previous ISBN 9780 9556 7465 5
e-ISBN 9781 4453 8588 4

**British Library Cataloguing-in-Publication Data**
A catalogue record for this book is available from
the British Library

Published by
BPP Learning Media Ltd
BPP House, Aldine Place
London W12 8AA

www.bpp.com/health

Typeset by Replika Press Pvt Ltd, India
Printed in the United Kingdom

ii

# Contents

*About the Publisher*
*About the Author*
*Acronyms and Abbreviations*
*Acknowledgements*
*Foreword*
*Preface*

**Section 1    The Interview as an Entity**

Chapter 1:    The context and philosophy of
the Consultant interview

Chapter 2:    Preparation prior to application:
do you feel ready?

Chapter 3:    Check your credentials and
apply

Chapter 4:    Research the Trust to which
you are applying before
shortlisting

Chapter 5:    Preparation after shortlisting:
the formal visit

Chapter 6:    Portfolio preparation, interview
practice and dress code

Chapter 7:    The Advisory Appointment
Committee (the interview
panel)

Chapter 8:    The presentation and other
pre-interview tasks

Chapter 9:    Performing on the day: your
body language, general
behaviour and influencing skills

**Section 2    Strategies**

Chapter 10:    Some general principles

Chapter 11:    Three vital principles

Chapter 12:    Questions investigating
self-reflection

Chapter 13:    Questions regarding scenarios

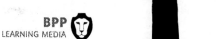

# About the Publisher

BPP Learning Media is dedicated to supporting aspiring professionals with top quality learning material. BPP Learning Media's commitment to success is shown by our record of quality, innovation and market leadership in paper-based and e-learning materials. BPP Learning Media's study materials are written by professionally-qualified specialists who know from personal experience the importance of top quality materials for success.

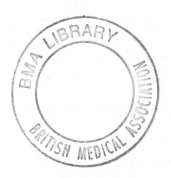

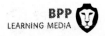

# About the Author

## Robert Ghosh

Robert Ghosh is a Consultant Physician at the Homerton University Hospital NHS Foundation Trust, London. He is the Clinical Director of Critical and Urgent Care, Director of Intensive Care, Clinical Lead for Acute Care and Chair of the Clinical Effectiveness and Audit Committee. He graduated from the University of Edinburgh, and his research interests include: the neuromuscular assessment of critically ill patients; prognostication in hypoxic brain injury; HIV test utilisation in poverty; and sedation scoring in critical illness. He has significant experience in interviewing for Consultant posts; he regularly provides guidance for prospective interviewees and continues to deliver courses on Consultant interviews on behalf of his company, Expertology Limited.

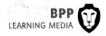

# Acronyms and Abbreviations

| | |
|---|---|
| AHCF | Academic Health Centres of the Future |
| ARCP | Annual Review of Competence Progression |
| BMA | British Medical Association |
| CaB | Choose and book |
| CCT | Certificate of Completion of Training |
| CFH | Connect for Health |
| CLRN | Comprehensive Local Research Network |
| CNST | Clinical Negligence Scheme for Trusts |
| COREC | Central Office for Research Ethics Committees |
| CQC | Care Quality Commission (this has also been referred to as 'Ofcare') |
| CQUIN | Commissioning for Quality and Innovation |
| DoH | Department of Health |
| ETP | Electronic transmission of prescriptions |
| EWTD | European Working Time Directive |
| GMC | General Medical Council |
| HaN | Hospital at night |
| HCC | Healthcare Commission |
| HRG | Healthcare resource groups |
| IBS | Indirectly bookable services |
| IRP | Independent review panel |
| IT | Information technology |
| LREC | Local Research Ethics Committees |
| LSP | Local Service Provider |
| MCA | Mental Capacity Act |
| MHRA | Medicines and Healthcare Products Regulatory Agency |
| MLCF | Medical Leadership Competency Framework |
| MMC | Modernising Medical Careers |
| MREC | Multi-centre Research Ethics Committees |
| NHS | National Health Service |
| NHS-MEE | NHS Medical Education England |
| NHSLA | NHS Litigation Authority |
| NICE | National Institute for Clinical Excellence |
| NIHR | National Institute for Healthcare Research |
| NIII | NHS Institute for Innovation and Improvement |

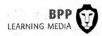

| | |
|---|---|
| NPfIT | National Project for Information Technology |
| NPSA | National Patient Safety Agency |
| NRLS | National Reporting and Learning System |
| NSP | National Service Provider |
| PACS | Picture Archiving and Communications System |
| PALS | Patient Advice and Liaison Services |
| PAS | Patient Administration System |
| PBR | Payment by results |
| PCT | Primary Care Trust |
| PLAB | Professional and Linguistic Assessment Board |
| PMETB | Postgraduate Medical Education and Training Board |
| QMAS | Quality Management Analysis System |
| RITA | Record of In-Training Assessment |
| SHA | Strategic Health Authority |
| SNOMED-CT | Systematised Nomenclature of Medicine Clinical Terms |
| STA | Specialist Training Authority |
| SUI | Serious untoward incident |
| UKCRN | UK Clinical Research Networks |
| WBR | Web-based referral |

# Acknowledgements

I would like to thank Angus, Bertie and Felicity for being the best, and Homerton University Hospital for nurturing me.

**Robert Ghosh**

## Crown Copyright

Many of the documents referred to in this book can be found on the Department of Health website (www.dh.gov.uk/en/Copyright/DH_4067693), and are reproduced here under the Open Government Licence (OGL).

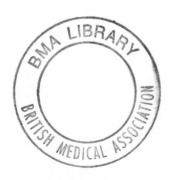

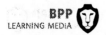

# Foreword

If you are reading this book the chances are that you are about to make the most important decision of your professional career ie where shall I work for the next 30 years? Your decision is pivotal in so much that you will spend a significant amount of your lifetime with your colleagues; even more so than with your partner and family. Your decision must also reflect the investment you have made in yourself over the course of your professional career. The Consultant interview may appear as a mountain, difficult and insurmountable. In reality the mountain is a mole hill and the most difficult question you must ask yourself is 'is this the correct job for me and do the people around the panel represent the people with whom I wish to spend the next 30 years?'

The Consultant interview requires preparation and as a fully trained professional you will be used to preparing for challenging events. In this book Robert Ghosh presents useful and relevant information to aid you in your approach and emphasises the need for preparation. The role of a Consultant is much wider than the role of Registrar, and as a trainee one is often not aware of the full range of duties required of a Consultant. Your preparation must include ensuring that you are educated in all the skills required and aware of the agenda of the National Health Service in general. Preparation for the interview itself requires knowledge of the Trust and of the people involved. The day of the interview looms large but again with preparation the height of the hurdle can be reduced. Think of the likely questions you may be asked and consider your responses using the methods suggested in this book. Only with practice can any skill be developed and honed.

A Consultant is a medical practitioner but also a leader and manager. The professional skills required of a Consultant are continually refined and developed. The interview panel will be aware of the stage you are at in your career and will ask you how you see your career developing. In this book Robert Ghosh has outlined many ways in which this may happen. The panel will not expect you to be an expert in all areas but to have an understanding of the problems faced by modern day Consultants and which areas of your skill base you feel require developing. After reading the

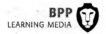

practical methods in this book, you can then consider the future development of your career and ensure that you can articulate your learning needs and what contribution your career plan will make to the Trust. Practise those answers, sound like a professional!

Any book is a living entity within a constantly changing world. I trust those of you who read this book and successfully complete the interview process will feed back to us the points that were useful and the points that need to be developed.

Good luck!

**Peter Livesley**
**MMed Sci (ClinEd) MCh Orth FRCS Orth**

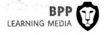

# Preface

It gives me great pleasure to once again write in this second edition of the interview book which deals with the pleasures, nuances and pitfalls for the prospective consultant interview candidate. There should be special mention to BPP Learning Media for initiating the momentum for updating, given the further radicalisation seen in healthcare over the last two to three years.

The main developments in this edition include some focus on psychometric assessments as adjuncts to interviews, the modernisation of out-dated nomenclature and historical facts, the addition of detailed quality agendas as 'hot topics' and the insertion of new seminal reports.

For those senior trainees, locum consultants and senior foreign doctors, the post of substantive consultant carries mixed images of established stereotypes, grandeur and an element of fear of the unknown with regard to modernisation in healthcare. It is true to say that the post remains the pinnacle in the eyes of most, notwithstanding the few who will aspire in future to be not only consultants but also clinical or executive directors. It is therefore paramount that every single potential interviewee gives the interview due respect; preparation should be meticulous.

Although most doctors do invest considerable time, effort and money in academic progression, it is probable that many do not spend the equivalent or sufficient time preparing for that all important Consultant interview. Most interviewees are eligible and skilled doctors who are well regarded by colleagues. They generally have the ability to build excellent relationships with patients. However, these attributes may not be apparent if the performance during the interview is below standard through lack of preparation.

Employers will look at new consultant recruits as leaders and valuable commodities, helping the institution deliver first class health care. They will need to see evidence of credibility, visible to patients and commissioners. They will also need to see evidence of teamworking which would sustain this credibility, rather than misplaced negativity or resistance.

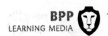

Selection criteria therefore, will be more stringent than ever; no longer will simple clinical credibility and tacit acknowledgement from ex-consultant bosses dictate success. Rather, the features of credibility and quality described in the paragraph above will need to shine in the presentation, the interview itself and also in any other (for example psychometric) assessments. Therefore preparation will be even more vital.

Particular attributes looked for in candidates are awareness of standards and leadership traits, and particular emphasis will be placed in this book on exactly these issues.

In this book, a few recommendations are dedicated to preparation prior to application, together with some advice on researching and visiting prior to shortlisting. The main remit however, is to help guide you, the prospective interviewee, through the interview process itself. This includes advice regarding: formal visits; presentations; interview behaviour traits; general principles for answers to commonly asked questions pertaining to factual knowledge, opinion and scenarios. It should be noted that presentations are increasingly (at time of writing) prominent, as healthcare institutions attempt to marry up the problem-solving preparation skills of the interviewee with their own needs.

Interviewers will inevitably take to candidates who possess the capacity for self-reflection, and who can handle clinical and non-clinical stressful situations. Moreover, as many on the panel will carry some of the Trust's burdens and anxieties, they will have an affinity for candidates who also have a sound working knowledge of the political landscape and common items on the trust's quality agenda. Therefore a great portion of this book contains summaries and questions related to these 'hot topics'.

Some chapters (particularly those relating to technique) are brief; on occasions they are not much more extensive than the summary page! This is a deliberate effort to keep things simple and reassure readers. The chapters relating to the hot topics are more traditional in size.

Specific detailed advice for academic appointments, for instance Senior Lecturer posts, is not within the remit of this book.

Although this book is not absolutely comprehensive, the information and guidance given here will hopefully go a long way towards equipping you with facts for preparation and insight into behavioural skills. I hope that this will in turn empower you to acquire the confidence to succeed.

Happy reading.

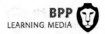

# Section 1

## The Interview as an Entity

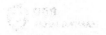

# Chapter 1

## The context and philosophy of the Consultant interview

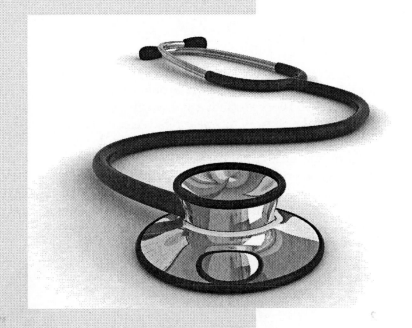

# The context and philosophy of the Consultant interview

Who or what is a Medical Consultant? An online medical dictionary refers to Medical Consultants as 'Individuals referred to for expert or professional advice or services'. Through the decades, definitions and contexts have changed. The role and duties of Consultants now encompass not only the authoritative and advisory aspect of clinical care, but also increasingly much of the day to day clinical care previously provided by junior doctors. In addition, the management duties previously delegated to other personnel have now (appropriately) come within their remit.

Some individuals may hark back to decades gone by, when the visiting Consultant would sweep into the gravel drive of a private hospital, be greeted by the Matron and taken into her room for tea, prior to conducting a ward round and thereby providing an opinion on the patients in the ward. More recently, salaried NHS Consultants continued to possess attractive work lifestyles – academic activities could easily be provided, job plans were often notional and very flexible, and clinical practice could be adapted to personal whims without financial or managerial recourse. Although much of the unmanaged flexibility has disappeared in the face of social and NHS modernisation, the job description and work/life balance of the Consultant continue to be very attractive and worth pursuing.

Most would agree that, in the face of social and NHS modernisation, the job description and work/life balance of the Medical Consultant continue to be very attractive and worth pursuing. Clinical activities continue to be a heady mix of applied science, hands-on intervention, social interaction with patients and colleagues, rapid action, cerebration, academia, camaraderie and authority. The pressures of Government and Trust targets, the need for more availability and concurrent requirement for management skills should all help create a more rounded approach to problem solving, and thereby create better doctors, and indeed better clinicians.

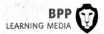

In modern, economically-driven healthcare policies, the post of Consultant is an asset which is becoming more measurable. This is particularly so during periods of economic hardship (and at time of writing we are in the midst of very difficult times). However, the measurability of assets is not oxymoronic with the subtleties of high profile, and you could argue that this simply brings the post of Consultant in line with other elite professions.

You should approach the commencement of Consultant duties, and therefore the Consultant interview, with excitement and relish. Unmitigated cynicism is a bad starting point, and should perhaps preclude application. This post should be seen as the pinnacle of your career.

There is no doubt that the value and relevance of the Consultant post is given immense respect by all those conducting the interview, and also by other senior personnel in the Trust to which the application is made. This respect, together with the obvious qualities of the job, should prompt the prospective interviewee to make meticulous preparations and treat the application and interview process with due consideration.

### Key points
You should:
- Absorb the history and know the importance of the job
- Realise that times have changed: this is not necessarily a bad thing
- Acknowledge the attributes and wide remit of the job
- Reflect on the so-called 'pressures': know that they generate responsibility, and help develop understanding
- Approach the job with enthusiasm and respect
- Be aware that this post is held in the highest regard by all senior personnel within the Trust

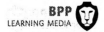

# Chapter 2

## Preparation prior to application: do you feel ready?

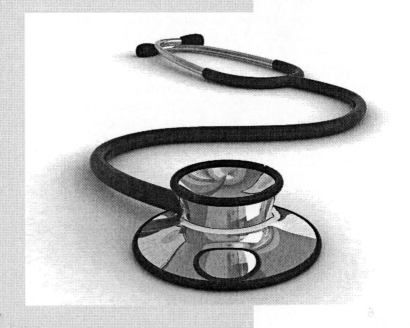

# Preparation prior to application: do you feel ready?

The vision and imagery of what it will be like to be an incumbent consultant should be clear. The highest level of clinical skills, the need for leadership, emotional intelligence, pragmatism and the possession of people-management skills are but some traits which the candidate should feel familiar with.

In these modern times, it is vital that Trusts not only survive but flourish. Commissioners will use the market economy to push institutions lacking in credibility into relative oblivion. These are the days when Trusts may need to fight for commissioners' recognition with other Trusts and indeed other organisations (such as private hospitals). It follows therefore that the employer will seek credibility and the candidate will need to demonstrate this.

It is true to say that the old fashioned values of standards cannot be entirely dismissed. The wise professor will attract custom, not least because the patients will want to be seen in a department with kudos. The candidate with a good research pedigree will carry the same type of attraction.

Contributing to Trust credibility by having an awareness of other visible and measurable standards, and teamworking skills to achieve corporate goals will be sought more and more in the interview. This is why a chapter in this book has been dedicated to the categorisation of standards. As mentioned in the previous chapter, the role of consultant is an asset which is becoming more and more measurable. I would yet again reinforce that this measurability does not negate the subtleties and elegance of the post.

Clearly the paperwork (namely the Deanery approval or other pathways to subsequent Specialist Registration, together with the Certificate or definite date for Specialist Registration) must be available at the time of the interview or within the acceptable time frame after the interview. However above all, you the candidate must 'feel ready'.

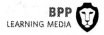

Your clinical skills should be exemplary, to the extent that you will have repeatedly provided a high quality clinical service without hands on supervision. This characteristic should be assumed as the norm, and will therefore be unlikely to separate the excellent candidates from the good ones in future interviews. The possession of sub-specialty skills may well impact, though they need to be relevant to the needs of the advertising Trust.

Most Consultants agree that it is non-clinical skills that separate good from average colleagues. Knowledge of up-to-date management and political topics is essential. For example, a sound knowledge of the NHS structure and relationships with Acute Trusts, an understanding of the makeup and responsibilities of the Trust Board, and an awareness of recent political issues and proposals will provide a basic framework within which to apply leadership skills. Subsequent chapters in this book will identify topics which you should be aware of, and which are commonly asked in interviews. Leadership qualities are needed daily and in particular at times of stress (to deal with angry colleagues, frustrated patients, resource shortcomings and so on). There is a fine line between authority and arrogance. There are several high quality management courses available; attendance of one of these will usually be mandatory prior to, or just after, appointment to a Consultant post.

Often, urgent or emergency advice will be sought from Consultants with regard to ethical dilemmas, rather than pure clinical challenges. You should be aware of current opinion. Seeking advice from a colleague is often a better option than procrastination. There is an increasing number of ethics and philosophy courses relevant to clinical medicine.

Your career up to this point should have equipped you with significant skills in multitasking and prioritisation in the clinical setting. As a Consultant, it is likely that these time management skills will more often be applied to management and other administrative duties. Successful audit, research and administrative activities as a trainee while in the midst of busy jobs should give a good impression.

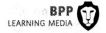

If you genuinely think that you have ticked these boxes and you 'feel ready', it is time to give the advertisement some serious consideration.

### Key points

You should:

- Possess a certificate or definite date for Specialist Registration
- Make sure your clinical skills are beyond reproach
- Be prepared to demonstrate credibility; credibility may be defined as the possession of academic/clinical prowess, or teamworking skills necessary to maintain the Trust's standing
- Be aware of management and political topics, and develop leadership skills; if necessary, attend an established course
- Be aware of ethical issues impacting on clinical decisions
- Develop time management skills and highlight examples in your CV

Above all, you must feel 'ready'.

# Chapter 3

## Check your credentials and apply

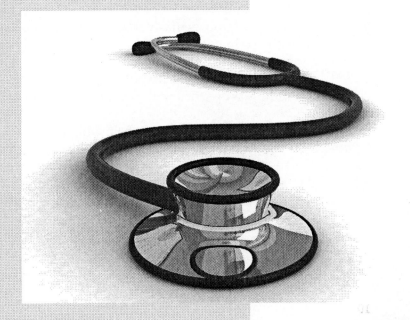

# Check your credentials and apply

Appointment criteria ('essential' and 'desirable') may be included in the job advertisement, and will certainly be prominently displayed in the job description. Possession of the entire essential (and at least some of the desirable) criteria on first reading of the job description is an essential starting point. If there is time to acquire an extra criterion prior to application, this is strongly recommended. For example, it is not uncommon for candidates to enrol and attend a worthwhile management course at very short notice. Sadly, many applicants are immediately rejected at the time of application as a result of not meeting the minimal requirements. This reflects badly on the applicant, who clearly has not understood or read the job description, and wastes the valuable time of those involved with shortlisting. A needless rejection will dent morale.

Almost all application forms will be available electronically; the applicant should give time and respect by typing the submission.

The details in the application and CV should tally. Neither should contain any discrepancies of fact. Common examples include incongruities of dates and chronology with regard to lists of previous posts and management, research and audit items included in the application, though not the CV (or vice versa). Be prepared to be asked about date gaps, particularly if you have not clarified this in your CV. These gaps in years gone by would universally be seen as a negative characteristic. Fortunately, philosophies have changed and it becomes the responsibility of the candidate to identify character- building properties within these periods of time.

There is a fine line between heavily embellishing your CV and lying. Judicious enhancement of facts (usually skills and experiences, particularly in the subjects of teaching, audit and research) is ethical; it is essential however, that this will sit comfortably in your own mind. Be prepared for meticulous dissection during the interview.

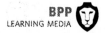

Candidates should be aware that some employers are increasingly using psychometric assessments not only as a pre-interview task but also in application forms. At time of writing it is less common to see the application of psychometrics in application than it is during the pre-interview episode. Readers should refer to the relevant pre-interview chapter in order to familiarise themselves with the principles of psychometric assessments.

## Key points

You should:

- Check your credentials against the appointment criteria: you should possess all the essential criteria and most or all of the desirable
- Consider achieving one more criterion at short notice eg a management course
- Type your application
- Include important details in both the application and the CV
- Check for discrepancies within your application form and CV, and between these documents (eg dates in posts)
- By all means, prominently display your skills in your CV, but do not over embellish, as you will be exposed in the interview
- Be aware that psychometric assessments may be occasionally used in application forms

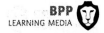

# Chapter 4

## Research the Trust to which you are applying before shortlisting

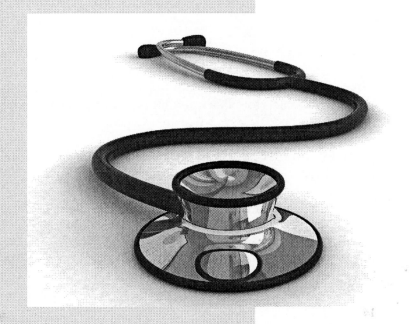

# Research the Trust to which you are applying before shortlisting

You will need to ensure that the Trust to which you are applying meets your requirements. Even if you have worked there in the past, there may have been recent changes to affect your working practice. It is important to note how your specialty or specialties are viewed by your potential colleagues, other medical personnel, non-medical staff, managers, the Trust Board, patients and the local Primary Care Trust. Do the personnel in the Department, Directorate and Trust have a reputation (good or bad) for anything in particular?

Much of this information may not be attainable without the time and diligence required from a formal post-shortlisting visit (see Chapter 5). However, informal opinions from junior doctors or other recent employees may be available to you.

All acute Trusts should have established internet/intranet sites. Considerable time and effort should be invested in researching the latter. Indeed the quality of the site itself may give you an impression of the quality (or lack) of information and visible priorities of the Trust. Take particular time to investigate the prominence and available information of your relevant Department and Specialty.

Other sources of important information include: the primary care trust website, the Strategic Health Authority website, and the Chief Medical Officer's Annual Report (there may be a section in that report which touches upon an issue, or clinical theme, which relates to the post).

If the information gathered so far is satisfactory, you may wish to consider visiting the Trust prior to shortlisting. It would be prudent to telephone or correspond with the Lead Clinician of the Department to establish whether this is acceptable. The aim of this *brief* visit is simply to absorb the atmosphere or 'flavour' of the hospital(s) and department(s), establish the nature of their location and facilities and confirm that you should proceed with

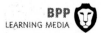

your application. Arranging formal appointments at this stage is not recommended.

### Key points

You should:

- Ensure that the Trust right for you
- Acquire information about how your specialty is seen by others within and outside the Trust
- Be aware of any reputations (good or bad) of the Department and/or Trust
- Visit the Trust's Internet/Intranet site
- Consider other sources of information
- Consider an informal visit if this acceptable with the Trust

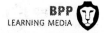

# Chapter 5

## Preparation after shortlisting: the formal visit

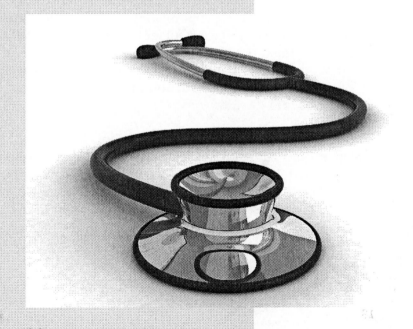

# Preparation after shortlisting: the formal visit

Hopefully, selection for interview will instil pride and excitement. Preparations should be made for a formal visit to the Trust, including all its hospital sites. It is true to say that anybody who does not visit the Trust/Department prior to their interview is seriously reducing their chances of success.

The purpose of the formal visit is not only to familiarise yourself with the panel, but most importantly also to acquaint yourself with the ongoing issues of the trust as seen through the eyes of key individuals. The information you will be given through your enquiries will greatly inform your strategy during the interview. It is clear therefore that you should not restrict the visit to individuals who are simply on the panel; if possible, key individuals who are able to offer a senior opinion of the trust should also be included.

Organise appointments with the Chief Executive, Medical Director, Clinical Director and Lead Clinician. If you have time, try and arrange to see the Directorate General Manager, the Departmental Lead Nurse or Matron, and key Executive Directors.

After the introductions, try to confirm your reasons for applying to the Trust, and also convey your interest in the strategic development and anxieties of Trusts. It is useful for key Trust individuals to know, even before the interview, that you take an interest in 'strategy', and that you would like to play a key role in 'development' and problem-solving, if appointed. You may be in a position to factor these issues into the interview.

During the visit, confirm the qualities and features of the Trust which prompted your application. The research described in Chapter 4 will have equipped you for this. It might also be helpful to find out the current research or special interests of relevant panel members, especially if the post is likely to bring you into professional contact with them.

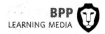

When questions are invited, it would be prudent to enquire from the Lead Clinician about the department's sub-specialty interests. There may be aspects that you were not aware of that are applicable to your skills and expertise. Questions pertaining to clinical shortfalls may also be directed to the Lead Clinician, though a different perspective to the same question may be provided by the Clinical Director. The Medical Director may have an opinion on perennial managerial problems with regard to the Department and the Trust. The Chief Executive is best placed to discuss the future direction and sensitive topics for the Trust.

When visiting the Department, take time to engage with all the relevant personnel. This may include nursing staff, physiotherapists, technicians and ward clerks. They may also have opinions and ideas about the satisfactory running of the department. Also, by visiting the departmental workforce you'll be seen as being an inclusive team player.

If you have made time to visit to the Directorate (Operational or 'General') Manager, you may find that (s)he has a unique non-medical perception on the running of the Department or Directorate. This may be important to you, and, if it is, you may wish to comment during the interview. In addition, the Departmental Modern Matron will be able to give you valuable insight into the issues facing your future nursing colleagues.

It may be relevant to visit key Executive Directors (other than the Chief Executive and Medical Director, who you will have already seen), who will have important opinions on strategic and topical issues. Their roles will include: Corporate Development; Planning; Service Development; Finance; Information; Nursing; Quality; Human Resources; Environment.

In posts which involve split sites, you should endeavour to visit all key personnel from all sites. If the sites are within the same Trust, it is likely that the extra visit will involve a satellite department. If the post encompasses more than one Trust, all the appointments mentioned above need to be replicated.

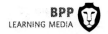

## Key points

You should:

- Organise appointments with the Chief Executive, Medical Director, Clinical Director and Lead Clinician
- Also try hard to arrange to see the Directorate General Manager, the departmental Lead Nurse/Matron, key Executive Directors and the departmental workforce
- Confirm the reasons for your application with the appropriate people and identify key issues:
  - Lead Clinician: Department's clinical interests
  - Clinical Director: clinical shortfalls
  - Medical Director: perennial managerial problems with regard to the Department and the Trust
  - Chief Executive: future direction and sensitive topics for the Trust
  - Department: engage with all relevant personnel
  - Directorate General Manager: non-medical perception of the Department or Directorate
  - Departmental Matron: issues for nurses
  - Key Executive Directors: strategic and topical issues
- Realise you may be able to give these key individuals the impression that you are a problem solver
- Realise you may be able to factor these issues into the interview
- Remember: split sites

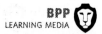

# Chapter 6

## Portfolio preparation, interview practice and dress code

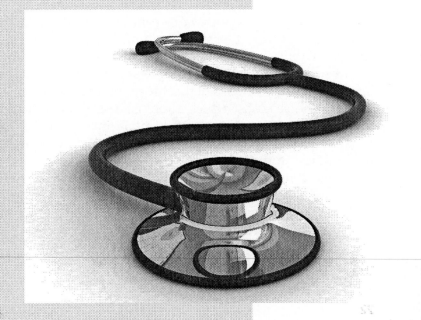

# Portfolio preparation, interview practice and dress code

## *Portfolio preparation*

Most candidates come to the interview equipped with their relevant logbook, if one exists. Most Royal Colleges, Deaneries or Learned Societies have templates or recommended formats available for downloading, and it is essential that this format is preserved, even if it is modified by individuals. Modification and expansion of the logbook to create a comprehensive portfolio is a novel idea, and an excellent one at that. This is best done electronically using spreadsheets, which may be printed out for perusal at the interview. Items dedicated per sheet (in addition to the logbook) may include experiences with: complaints; risk; business cases; difficult clinical situations; situations leading to a change in practice; ethical dilemmas encountered; situations requiring leadership skills; situations requiring management skills; and attendance or response to external visits from relevant bodies. If questions on these matters are asked during the interview, an articulate response from the candidate may be accompanied by an invitation to the panel to read the relevant item in the portfolio.

## *Interview practice*

The value of interview practice cannot be underestimated. It is recommended that at least two willing Consultant colleagues are identified, though it may initially be useful to run mock interviews with a single interviewer. The venue should be quiet and free from interruptions. It is important that the candidate prepares thoroughly prior to the sessions, which should be taken seriously by both the mock interviewer and mock interviewee. The pre-prepared questions should be asked professionally, and the answers should be delivered in the manner you would expect to see at the actual interview. It may be useful to undergo a final mock interview near the actual day; this would preferably involve two interviewers, with the interviewee having (hopefully) prepared more fully, and perhaps attired formally.

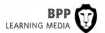

## *Dress code*

Dress is mainly a social signal. In day-to-day life it informs others of your style, status and social grouping. Although there is no 'dress code' and the attire is largely a matter of personal choice, you should attempt to conform to the norms of the people you are trying to influence, namely the panel. You should therefore appear formal, smart and professional and the clothes must feel comfortable. Dark suits are preferable for both men and women. Skirts and trousers are equally acceptable for women. You should be wary of accessories, for example cufflinks for men and earrings and necklaces for women. These should not attract more attention than you do. Try to avoid wearing items such as club ties which have a chance of provoking tribalism. Ensure your shoes are polished and clean. Avoid unnecessary strong smells – such as pungent after-shave/perfume, strong cooking odours or cigarette smoke.

## Key points

**Portfolio preparation**
- Come equipped with the relevant logbook
- Consider modifying and expanding the logbook to create a comprehensive portfolio
- Be aware of key topics such as: complaints; risk; business cases; difficult clinical situations; situations leading to a change in practice; ethical dilemmas encountered; situations requiring leadership skills; situations requiring management skills; and attendance or response to external visits from bodies such as the Care Quality Commission

**Interview practice is highly recommended**
- Prepare thoroughly
- Interview practice should be taken seriously by both the mock interviewer and mock interviewee

**Dress code**
- Dress formally and ensure that you are smart, professional and comfortable
- Avoid tribalism
- Avoid distracting accessories
- Avoid pungent aftershave/perfume and spicy food

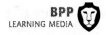

# Chapter 7

## The Advisory Appointment Committee (the interview panel)

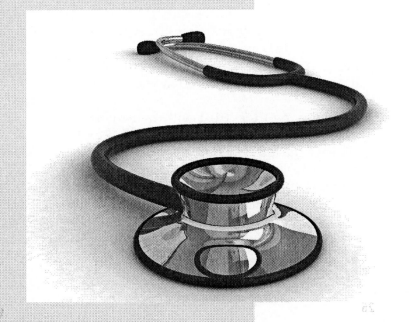

# The Advisory Appointment Committee (the interview panel)

The technical role of the Advisory Appointment Committee (AAC) is to *recommend*, via a shortlisting and interview process, one or more suitable candidates *to the Trust (Executive Board)*. In reality, the AAC is given delegation responsibilities to make this decision on behalf of the Trust. The interview itself, although normally held in a standard format, will occasionally occur via video link if this is the most practical method. The AAC must be present in any format.

Guidelines and conventions suggest that *at least* the following six individuals should sit on the panel:

1. Chief Executive Officer
2. Medical Director
3. Consultant
4. Royal College representative (not essential in Foundation Trusts, though is still advised)
5. University representative (in posts with formal teaching and/or research duties)
6. Lay member (usually the Chairman of the Trust)

In reality the panel will be larger, as described in this chapter. Indeed it is likely that this will be your first interview where the numbers making up the panel are so large. Each individual panellist will have an important role to play, and their questions will be relevant to their experience and their role.

The Chairman of the Trust will chair the proceeding. He or she is likely to introduce him/herself and the other panellists, and commence the interview process by confirming your identity, and asking some benign questions pertaining to the CV. The Chief Executive Officer will most often concentrate on concepts of vision, strategy, management, leadership and self-reflection. The Medical Director may focus on perennial medical problems affecting the Trust. This may or may not have direct relevance to your specialty.

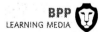

There will often be a focus on revalidation, appraisal, probity and data protection. The Clinical Director may have a similar approach to, and type of questions as, the Medical Director.

It is more likely that any management or strategy question, for instance Government targets, will have relevance to the Department and Directorate. The External College Representative is there to provide an external view of previous training, practice development and general competency. He or she may enquire about any clinical shortfalls in your development or training thus far. You should be aware that although Foundation Trusts often do include college representatives at their interviews, they are not obliged to do so. The Lead Clinician is there as a potential close colleague, and will therefore see him/herself as a gatekeeper for the Department. It may be here that your logbook and sub-specialty skills come under the closest scrutiny; visions for progress of the Department may be asked for. There will be a University Representative if the post is an academic appointment. In addition, more and more District General Hospitals are now University Hospitals, and therefore university representation is required at these interviews. Some questions may be directed at undergraduate teaching. The Human Resources representative is unlikely to ask any questions during the body of the interview, and will ask questions on eligibility and commencement date at the end.

In split site posts there may be duplication of key personnel from other sites.

Increasingly there are lay people on the panel representing patient and community perspectives. They are there to provide a non-medical stakeholder viewpoint. It is particularly important therefore that your responses to questions are pitched correctly, that you take into account the varying level of technical understanding of all panel members, and display empathy for patients and relatives in all your answers.

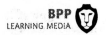

**Key points**

You should be aware that the AAC (interview panel) is large and each individual has a specific role:

- Chairman: makes introductions and chairs the interview panel
- Chief Executive Officer: often asks about vision, strategy and leadership
- Medical Director: often asks about revalidation, appraisal, probity and data protection
- Clinical Director: often asks about quality indicators including finance
- External College Representative: ensures quality assurance for previous training and competencies
- Lead Clinician: gatekeeper for the department; often asks about clinical skills and vision for the department
- University Representative (if relevant): teaching and research
- Human Resources
- Representatives from other sites in split site posts
- Lay individual

# Chapter 8

## The presentation and other pre-interview tasks

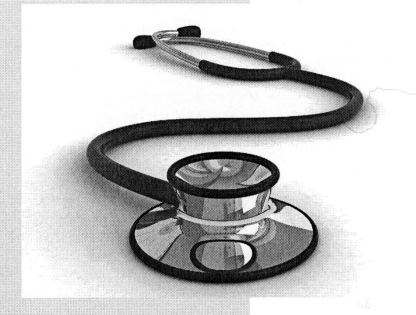

# The presentation and other pre-interview tasks

Having mentioned more than once in previous chapters the importance of teamwork with regard to Trust goals and standards, it should come as no surprise that pre-interview presentations and other tasks are primarily designed to map these attributes, and are increasingly prevalent before interviews. The main task presented to interviewees before the interview itself in addition to the presentation is a collection of 'stations' (similar to medical exams) where problems are presented and psychometrics are applied. It is more vital than ever that candidates are aware of what employers are looking for in these pre-interview tasks.

This chapter will concentrate on the presentation and a brief description of the 'stations'.

When employers construct presentation tasks for prospective candidates, they are assessing the ability of these candidates to: understand the question; apply context to recent political developments and ongoing issues; invariably map the answers to topics relating to *standards and goals*; understand in detail the method of presentation; and present with efficiency and genuine feeling.

Presentations take on many formats, some being more common than others. The formats less frequently employed may become more prevalent in the years to come.

The time of day and duration set aside for the presentation is also not consistent. More often, a half day will be set aside for the candidates to present individually to the panel. Alternatively, the opportunity to present will arise during the interview session itself.

The most common state of affairs is that the topic and audio-visual format will be pre-determined by the Trust, and identified for the candidate significantly in advance. This topic may relate to: your vision for the Department/Trust; how you can help the Trust develop; improving clinical effectiveness in your specialty; the future (and

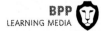

controversies) of your specialty; assessing clinical performance in your specialty. When preparing for the presentation, you should consider not only the simple processes involved in achieving the endpoints associated with the topic, but also the relevance of local pressures on the Trust. You may therefore consider: the usage of clinical audit as a tool to improve quality and clinical effectiveness; Trust quality ratings; and patient-centred themes.

These are some fictional examples:

**As part of the interview you will be required to provide a 15-minute/30-minute/45-minute presentation addressing the following topic:**

*'Describe ways in which standards are measured in your specialty, and how you can use these to locally maintain clinical excellence'.*

*OR*

*'Describe ways in which you could use risk to improve your department's quality.'*

*OR*

*'Describe ways in which you could measure patient experience outcomes in your department.'*

*OR*

*'Describe ways in which financial measurements in your department could improve quality'.*

*Please email a maximum of 5 slides / 10 slides / 15 slides (A4 – typeset a minimum of 16 using Microsoft Word or PowerPoint) which we will print onto acetates for you to use with an overhead projector (not by PowerPoint projection) as part of your presentation – these slides could include diagrams, key points you would like to get across etc. You will also be expected to answer any questions arising from your presentation – the latter may take up to 15 minutes.*

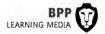

From the instructions above it is clear that the presentation must not exceed the time limitation and the slides will be printed onto acetates. Therefore you should ensure that your talk flows consistently without the aided technology of PowerPoint; the topic should be stated clearly.

When preparing your presentation it is important that it has an introduction, a main section and a conclusion. When performing a presentation it is important to: introduce yourself and the topic you are going to talk about; provide background or context to the approach you have taken in preparing your presentation; and ensure that the main section, and indeed the presentation overall, clearly answers the question or explains your chosen topic.

Some common pitfalls are: missing a core relevant issue; not addressing the question or issue that has been requested; talking too quickly; overrunning on the stipulated time; not speaking loudly or clearly enough; not facing the audience and engaging them; unclear slides; too much information on the slides; using jargon, abbreviations or acronyms; and not being equipped to answer questions arising from your presentation.

Less commonly, although the topic is announced in advance, the audio-visual format may not be. This strategy is designed to identify the candidates who will have prepared their thoughts on the subject, and have the ability to modify their delivery. The principles of preparation and pitfalls are similar to those described above.

Rarely, neither the topic nor the audio-visual format is announced until the day of the presentation and interview. For instance, the candidate may be left on the day with an instruction for the topic, together with a flipchart and pens. The purpose of this exercise is to select the candidate with the ability to rapidly identify the reason behind the selection of the topic by the Trust, the salient issues, the possible controversies and also the most efficient method of delivery.

You should remember that even if the presentation has a clinical theme, there are almost always non-clinical topics which the employers will wish to see mentioned.

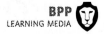

For example, if the title of the presentation is 'laparoscopic colorectal surgery', it is a virtual certainty that the topics of patient satisfaction, length of stay, finance and quality indicators will need to be factored in.

Employers will often set up 'scenario stations' as a vehicle for psychometric tasks. Indeed, psychometric tasks are occasionally used in the written application process. The history of this type of tactic comes from military recruitment, and more recently from industry recruitment. Psychometric tests often highlight personality and behaviour traits which could be seen to be more conducive to teamworking. It should be pointed out that sadly it is not uncommon for employers to simply see psychometric tests as advantageous in themselves without grasping the concept that the tests need to be applicable to the post and context. A badly selected psychometric test will inevitably select at best an irrelevant candidate and at worst the wrong candidate. A properly selected psychometric test will deal with the following, among other things:

- Generic leadership skills
- Assertiveness/submissiveness
- Respect for the team and individuals' roles
- Tendency to frustration and anxiety/appropriate calmness
- Articulation and general teamworking skills
- Appropriate risk-taking for the benefit of the department/Trust

Many employers may choose to assess these generic attributes without applying them to relevant contexts (for example generic questionnaires). However, it is a more successful strategy to apply psychometric assessments to scenarios. Although it is not rare for psychologists to be used during these 'stations', it is more common for members of the interview panel (who should be competent assessors) to perform the assessment.

It is extremely important that candidates do not try to 'second-guess' the correct results for psychometric tests, whether the format is written (for applications) or verbal. This will inevitably lead to a misrepresentation of yourself, and this in turn will not serve you well. A much better strategy is for you to be yourself, and take the consequences.

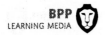

'Scenario stations' may include any of the scenarios that are described in this book. There is not a huge difference between the traditional approach of the panel assessing your response to a scenario question, and observers assessing your response in a station closer to a 'real life' situation. Psychometric tests are more easily applied in the latter.

## Key points

**Presentations are increasingly common. Be aware of:**

- The agenda: a half-day may be set aside for the presentation, or it may be incorporated into the interview
- Varying formats: pre-set topic with audio-visual format necessitates an awareness of local pressures on the Trust; pre-set topic, with audio-visual format determined on the day necessitates sound preparation and flexible delivery; topic and audio-visual format determined on the day necessitates rapid identification of the reason for topic selection and delivery method
- Common pitfalls

**Psychometric testing (mock scenario) stations are increasingly common.**

- Be aware of the aims: they are designed to highlight behaviour and personality traits which are conducive with team working; they often deal with leadership skills, assertiveness, submissiveness, tendency to frustration and anxiety, articulation and general team working skills
- Never 'second-guess' in psychometric testing – always be yourself

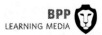

# Chapter 9

**Performing on the day: your body language, general behaviour and influencing skills**

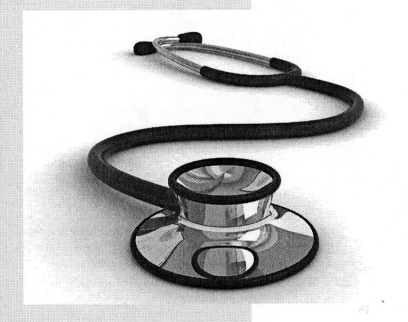

# Performing on the day: your body language, general behaviour and influencing skills

It is important to acknowledge that *confidence* will influence how you behave on the day, and how you conduct yourself during the interview will play a large role in success or failure, irrespective of your preparations thus far. You must assume that you are at least on par with your competitors. 'I am not the preferred candidate' is a commonly quoted grievance. It should therefore be noted that the 'internal' candidate may not be preferred, or may interview very badly. Often there is no preferred candidate at all. You should believe that the interview is a level playing field.

It is important to have learnt from previous interviews, particularly if you have received feedback from the panel. Address those issues and do not repeat previous mistakes.

Panellists will judge you by your behaviour. They do not know you, and even if the behaviour you show on the day is an aberration, they will not be able to differentiate this from your true self. Although difficult, the influential traits to try and put across are: flexibility (pragmatism where two choices in the solution to a problem may conflict); generosity (manifested in conversation); trustworthiness (demonstrated in response to questions); persistence in pursuit of goals (though not to the point of futility); optimism (though not blind – demonstrated in response to questions); and an analytical approach (careful reasoning in response to questions). In matters of debate it is important to display reasoning skills without arguing as the latter will build up resistance among the panellists. As it is likely that you will be one of several candidates, it is important to stand out without seeming overly quirky. The best and most efficient way of achieving this other than possessing sheer credibility is to display the influential characteristics described above better than your competitors.

It is good practice to visualise the impression you want to make (for example assertiveness, competence, reliability and leadership). You should then plan for it, taking into account your mannerisms and behaviour. Never, however be false – always be true to yourself.

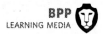

Many experts recommend that you internally visualise the interview. If the mere thought of the big day feels you full of dread, re-enact the scene in your mind until you feel you have ironed out potential problems. Perpetually re-enact the scene until you feel you have perfected your strategy, and you have created that perfect, successful scene. It is a possibility that your behaviour at the interview and your confidence will be linked to this mental image. Positive thoughts (for example looking forward to meeting you future colleagues) should reinforce this mental image. It is important to remember that complete obliteration of nerves is a false outcome and should not be strived for, as it is recognised that a little bit of nerves heightens performance.

Body language is worth practising, even in front of the mirror. First impressions count and behaviours can be adapted while remaining true to oneself – remember, never be false.

The two main attributes which heighten rapport are eye contact and smiling. Making eye contact is very important for reinforcing genuineness – this includes acknowledging the panel on entry to the room. You should avoid prolonged spells of looking away from the questioner at the floor and at the ceiling. It is also important not to concentrate on making eye contact solely with the questioner; this will give the impression of monopolising the conversation with one person, whereas intermittent eye contact with the rest of the panel will make them feel included. Smiling should be natural; false, derived smiles can be unnerving. Other general features emphasising calmness and confidence include walking with steady, non-hesitant strides and with an erect posture.

When you sit down, make sure that you maintain the body language of assertion and confidence. You should be relaxed and professional. Over-relaxation to the point of slouching will be interpreted as slackness and unprofessionalism. There are many different favoured seating positions, and you must choose the position that suits you most. Most sit upright with hands placed comfortably on the lap. Most agree that both feet should be on the floor.

Our hands are the most obvious signal of our nerves. You should avoid fiddling and making too many gestures (for example, pointing). Try to avoid crossing your arms, as virtually everyone

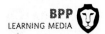

agrees that this is a defensive posture. You may wish to take simple steps to avoid bad habits on the day of the interview (for example you may choose not to wear jewellery which you always fiddle with).

The volume and depth of your voice and speed of speech delivery is worth a mention. It is a good idea to record yourself for practice. Within the constraints of your normal voice characteristics, the volume should be neither too loud nor too soft and the depth should not be too high or too low. In striving for neutral volume and depth, confidence and gravitas is often associated with a voice which has sufficient audibility and depth. The speed of delivery should provide clarity. The volume, depth and character of your voice should match the content of your conversation, whether you are being enthusiastic or thoughtful. Whether the sentences should be long, detailed or brief depends on the nature of the conversation; you should be prepared to take your cue from the panel. It will often be obvious when they want you to stop speaking. You should make every attempt to use the panellists' names – this should display genuine interest in the panel. It is good practice to demonstrate genuine interest in the question when applicable. One technique which often reinforces rapport is matching language choices to the questioner's; re-using some key words or phrases may demonstrate empathy. It is vital that this is not overdone as blatant mimicking will be insulting to the questioner.

The final pointer is the recommendation that once you have created that perfect scene and incorporated the advice in this chapter, you should above all maintain spontaneity and not appear as if you are robotically following a protocol.

 **Key points**

- Confidence will influence how you will behave on the day
- How you behave on the day will play a large role in the outcome
- Learn from previous attempts
- Influential traits include flexibility, generosity, trustworthiness, persistence, optimism and an analytical approach
- Try to stand out without seeming quirky
- Consider internally visualising the interview and repeating the scene until it is perfect

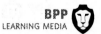

- Assess and practise body language traits, particularly eye contact and smiling
- Assess and practise seating posture, particularly hand posture
- Assess and practise speech: volume and depth of voice, speed of delivery, and length of answers
- *Consider* using the panellists' names when appropriate
- *Consider* matching language choices
- When following the above advice always be spontaneous, *not robotic*

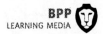

# Section 2

## Strategies

# Chapter 10
## Some general principles

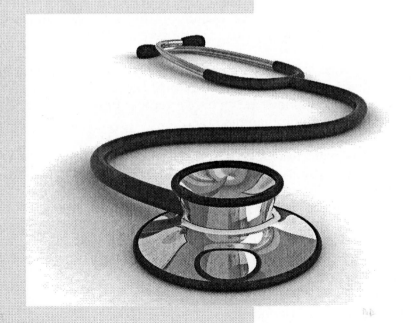

# Some general principles

## *Focus on non-clinical issues*

It is not surprising that many questions asked in Consultant interviews centre on topics pertaining to management, leadership and non-clinical attributes. Your future employers and the panel will take your clinical skills for granted, though they will want to be reassured that your awareness of national management politics, Trust infrastructure and perennial anxieties are sound. The latter may include financial principles, maintenance of standards, external checks for standards, risk, complaints, legal issues and ethical considerations.

## *Leave an impression and focus on language skills*

It is most important to remember that the interviewers, during the brief 40-minute period, want to get to know you. Are you what they want in a colleague? Well thought-out and articulate answers to difficult questions should give them the impression that you are a good problem-solver, which would be an asset to the Department. You should inwardly dissect the reason why the question has been asked; among other things, the panel may be seeking evidence of self-reflection, truthfulness or priorities. Once this is clear, it should be a little bit easier to give the interviewers what they want to hear. Identifying the reasoning behind a question will be a recurring theme in this book.

Answers should be brief, relevant and should wholly answer the question. This may seem obvious, however, it is not uncommon to find candidates being either verbose or too brief. The former is more common than the latter.

Most candidates recall successful interviews as a series of conversations, rather than an interrogation. Taking this notion further, the candidate may feel that (s)he is providing valuable, factual information in addition to the required answer, and that this information is being appreciated by the panel. Pleasant, lengthy discussions should not be confused with protracted questioning by the panel in the event of the candidate blatantly not grasping the point of the question!

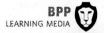

It is important that the tone of your answers indicate your respect for the panel members and the questions they put to you. However, it is equally important not to sound apologetic. Avoid using phrases such as 'You know' and 'As I previously said' which may be construed to be condescending by the panel.

Always seek to go beyond simply providing a 'textbook' reply. Many candidates do not appreciate that their 'parrot' answers are easily apparent to interviewers. The panel is keen to learn about *you*, rather than your recollection skills.

## Be sure of your declared expertise

It is also important to note that any information (for instance expertise in a particular field, such as teaching or research) that is presented in your CV or fashioned into the interview in the form of an answer can become the focus of detailed, in-depth questioning by the interview panel. Therefore it is essential that you do not choose to raise topics that you are not extremely confident about.

## Have an opinion but do not be opinionated

Even if you are extremely sure of your ground, the interview is not the forum to express controversial views on a particular subject. You need to strike a balance between demonstrating independent thought and presenting a solid, professional opinion. You need to show that you are an individual personality, yet also someone who can fit into a team and conform to the required standard of conduct.

## Use the introductory questions to settle your nerves

After completing the introductions and putting you at ease, the Chairman may begin with some initial questions, which are likely to be introductory and benign in nature. They are not designed to be taxing, and are unlikely to differentiate between interview success and failure. The questions may simply seek to confirm your credentials with the aid of your CV. Alternatively, there may be open introductory questions or requests such as 'Why did you apply for this post?' or 'Tell us something about yourself'.

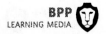

There may be specific questions arising from your presentation. Clearly, preparation and research around the topic should have been performed before the day of presentation, and therefore the questions should not be unpredictable. For the 'ad hoc' presentations, you should make time to organise your thoughts after the performance, in preparation for questions on the topic or even your method of presentation.

Ensuing questions may be categorised into:

- Those relating to fact, where an explanation or understanding is sought
- Those relating to opinion
- An assessment of the candidate's approach, often by way of a scenario

## Indentify the questions relating to fact

Simple factual questions are relatively uncommon, for instance, 'Could you tell me something about the NHS plan?' Here, the interviewer is simply asking for a brief demonstration of your working knowledge. It is more common for there to be some relevance to topical issues or your specialty, and you should take your cue from the interviewer before expanding on this. For instance, a more likely question may be 'Has the NHS Plan delivered for diabetes?'

## Be pragmatic with the questions on opinion

Questions on opinions are fairly frequent and are traditionally answered badly, for example, 'What is your opinion on junior doctors' training?' The aim here is to demonstrate your identification of pros and cons and then arrive at a pragmatic and wise conclusion. There is almost never a 'right' or 'wrong' answer. If you choose to firmly commit to a certain view, you should be aware that there will inevitably be individuals on the panel who will disagree, and there is the risk that the whole panel will disapprove of the lack of pragmatism.

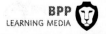

## *Navigate through the scenario questions*

In 'approach' and 'scenario' questions, you should rapidly identify the issue or problem. You may wish to demonstrate your methodology with a short introductory explanation, for example, 'I believe this is a question of professional/criminal conduct' or 'I believe this is a question of ethics'. In relevant questions you should be aware of the processes involved eg for the risk management system, complaints and fitness for practice. You would do well to remember that most roads lead to patient safety and welfare. These principles also apply to psychometric analyses at stations.

### Key points

- Focus on non-clinical issues – particularly management, leadership, finance, standards, risk, complaints, law and ethics
- Leave an impression and focus on being articulate; the interviewers want to get to know you
- Be sure of your declared expertise: any information that you give in the form of an answer may become the focus of detailed, in-depth questioning from the panel
- Have an opinion but do not be opinionated
- Use the introductory questions to settle your nerves
- Identify the questions relating to fact: these require a brief demonstration of working knowledge – these are commonly relevant to topical issues or your specialty
- Be pragmatic with the questions on opinion
- Navigate through the scenario questions: identify the issue or problem

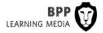

# Chapter 11

## Three vital principles

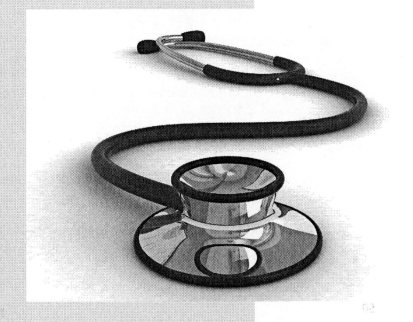

# Three vital principles

This chapter is deliberately very brief. The isolation of these principles is intended to highlight their importance, and to give you an opportunity to remember to apply these principles for the questions in the following chapters.

## *Know your standards*

As mentioned in previous chapters, the topic of standards is most likely to make itself known in interview questions in various guises. The employer will want to ensure that the candidate possesses the attributes to underpin the way that standards are measured by the employer and the employer's stakeholders. Indeed, standards are so important it is most likely that they will form the basis of most of the questions and also the presentation. 'All questions must be brought back to standards'. Although it is true to say that there are many ways of categorising standards, there should be a systematic approach to how you analyse standards for your own behaviour and specialty, to help clarify the background to questions and therefore strategies for answers.

You can begin by identifying the source of standards for you and your specialty. The origins may stem from the Department of Health, strategic health authorities (or equivalent), commissioners, governors, the trust (by way of committee) or your department. You must not forget professional standards as set out by bodies such as the General Medical Council and also those highlighted by other stakeholders such as other professional groups (for example nurses and physiotherapists), medical colleagues including general practitioners and patients. It may be practical separating out clinical standards from non-clinical ones. Clinical standards may include those of performance as measured by the job plan, those expected by your national specialty body and those expected by your employer. All these need to be underpinned by satisfactory continuing professional development (CPD) episodes. Non-clinical standards may also include those of performance and mainly tend to be those expected by your employer. It is a worthwhile exercise to try to associate as many interview questions as possible with the notion of standards.

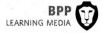

## *Identify different ways of asking the same question*

There are often different ways of asking the same question. For example: 'What qualities can you bring to the Trust/Department?'; 'What are your greatest strengths?'; 'What do you have to offer us?'; and 'Why should we recruit you rather than any of the other candidates?' are all asking for differentiating qualities when compared with others. 'Tell us about the two most recent NICE guidelines relating to your specialty. Did you and your department adopt them? Why/why not?' and 'Should we always adopt NICE guidelines?' both examine the process of putting evidence into practice. In the ensuing chapters, try to group together the questions which you feel should generate a similar response.

## *Make your answer relevant to your specialty*

Always attempt to highlight the relevance of your answer to your specialty and the interviewing Trust. For instance, general questions relating to quality or performance, and the Care Quality Commission, may be seeking an answer dealing with your knowledge of the roles of the CQC and consequent pressures on Trusts, the specific visits or issues relating to your specialty, your personal involvement with these issues and your ideas on improvement in quality and performance. Other examples include the National Patient Safety Agency, Strategic Health Authorities and Payment by Results. Be aware that your answer, if of sufficient quality, will give the panel the impression that you may have the knowledge, insight and solutions to many of the Trust's problems and anxieties.

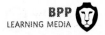

### Key points

You should adopt these principles for the relevant questions in the following chapters:

- Assume that virtually all questions are linked to standards. Be aware of the various sources and stakeholders. Develop a way of categorising standards in your specialty and for yourself. It is a worthwhile exercise to try to associate as many interview questions as possible with the notion of standards
- There are often different ways of asking the same question. In the ensuing chapters, try to group together the questions which you feel should generate a similar response
- Particularly in response to questions on quality or performance (eg Care Quality Commission, Payment by Results), try to attempt to highlight the relevance of your answer to your specialty and the interviewing Trust. Be aware that your answer, if of sufficient quality, will give the panel the impression that you may have the knowledge, insight and solutions to many of the Trust's problems and anxieties

# Chapter 12

## Questions investigating self-reflection

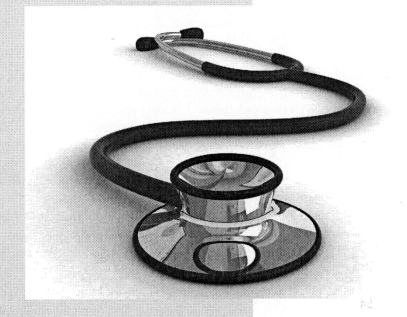

# Questions investigating self-reflection

The interview panel may try to reveal your virtues and weaknesses, perhaps by asking about them directly, or by asking about your aptitudes and ambitions. Answers tend to reveal your personal values. Questions about weaknesses, mistakes, tasks that you could have done better or opportunities missed, set out to measure your self-awareness, intellectual honesty, maturity and dependability; they may also highlight your team membership characteristics. The panel will wish to identify particular aspects and attributes. Issues of leadership and credibility are paramount.

When identifying issues of leadership, it should be recognised that the definition of leadership can mean many things to different people. Many doctors will volunteer the notion that 'we cannot all be leaders'. Although this may be true without delving into semantics too much, it should be appreciated that if one definition of leadership is 'to be able to influence', you should aspire to this. Questions may therefore be directed toward influential qualities. We will go into a little more detail on leadership qualities later on in this chapter.

As mentioned before (and will be mentioned again), the topic of credibility is key. You may ooze credibility on the basis of your research and clinical pedigree, or on the basis of managerial skills mapping to the requirements of the employers. Questions will be directed to highlight these issues.

Questions about your greatest achievements, challenges or responsibilities are an attempt to obtain a record of your standards. Your challenge may be to identify those which may be more prominent than the average doctor, and indeed more prominent than your competitor candidates. These may include crisis management qualities, negotiation skills or leadership style. Questions about relationships are trying to assess your personality: are you social or self-contained, conforming or independent, extrovert or sensitive, phlegmatic or excitable?

There are no 'correct' answers to many of the questions in this chapter.

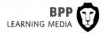

## Relevant questions – application

1. Tell us the reasons for applying for this post.
2. Why do you want to join our Trust?
3. What concerns you about this job?
4. What do you think will be your biggest challenge in this post?
5. What are you hoping to gain from this post?

These questions are designed to encourage the candidate to reflect on the benefits and drawbacks of the post; this may include issues with the region (poverty, affluence and aged population), the Trust (tertiary services, special attributes), the Department (size, special attributes) or clinical duties (sub-specialty skills at which you are particularly capable). It should be obvious to the panel that the challenges and drawbacks are not in your eyes insurmountable – after all you have attended the interview! Nevertheless you should articulately clarify your plans to deal with the challenges.

## Relevant questions – specialty

1. Which attributes of this specialty made you choose it?
2. What are the challenges or controversies in your specialty?
3. Why did you choose to follow a career in this specialty?
4. If you were to start your career again, what would you change?
5. Why do you want to pursue this specialty?
6. What do you dislike about your chosen specialty?
7. How would you dissuade a colleague from entering your specialty?
8. What are the challenges facing this specialty over the next ten years?
9. What steps have you taken throughout your career to confirm this is the right career choice for you?

The panel is attempting to obtain a fuller picture of the candidate. The challenges may be national and topical or local (see above). As the candidate has progressed to this level, any dislikes of the candidate's speciality are clearly minor. The 'dissuading' question identifies the candidate who has the ability to recognise the

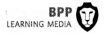

drawbacks of the specialty and correlate this with the profile of the colleague. After performing this exercise you may wish to reassure the panel that the drawbacks are not relevant to you.

## Relevant questions – qualities

1. What qualities can you bring to the Trust/Department?
2. What is your greatest achievement?
3. What are your greatest strengths?
4. What do you have to offer us?
5. Why should we recruit you rather than any other candidate?
6. What makes you a good candidate for the job?
7. What three adjectives describe you best?
8. What would your friends say about you?
9. What are your ambitions as a doctor?
10. Where do you see yourself in 2 years' / 5 years' / 10 years' time? What is your ambition as a Consultant?
11. What skills have you gained that will make you a good doctor?
12. What are the qualities of a good doctor?
13. What kind of feedback would I obtain from your patients if I asked them?
14. How do you measure success in your field?
15. Would you be happy being an average Consultant?

When asked about qualities, achievements and strengths, it would be prudent to remember that many candidates will give stock answers and may simply give an answer 'expected of a Registrar'. You will need to identify strengths that are unlikely to be shared (or spotted) by the other candidates, qualities which would make you an above average senior doctor (for example leadership and management skills) and those abilities particularly relevant to the pressures on the Trust or Department (gleaned from your formal visits).

Questions on self-description are intended to highlight self-reflection, and should give the panel an idea of the type of person you are. Avoid simply singing your own praises.

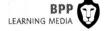

Remember that ambition may relate to career or personal issues. The former in turn should involve visions for the specialty, the Department and the Trust.

The philosophy of 'being a good doctor' is well encapsulated in the General Medical Council's guidelines which describe the duties of a doctor within the UK (www.gmc-uk.org/guidance/good_medical_practice/duties_of_a_doctor.asp):

- Make the care of your patient your first concern
- Treat every patient politely and considerately
- Respect patients' dignity and privacy
- Listen to patients and respect their views
- Give patients information in a way that they can understand
- Respect the rights of patients to be fully involved in decisions about their care
- Keep your professional knowledge and skills up to date
- Recognise the limits of your professional competence
- Be honest and trustworthy
- Respect and protect confidential information
- Make sure that your personal beliefs do not prejudice your patients' care
- Act quickly to protect patients from risk if you have good reason to believe that you or a colleague may not be fit to practise
- Avoid abusing your position as a doctor
- Work with colleagues in the ways that best serve the patients' interests
- In all situations you must never discriminate unfairly against your patients and colleagues and must always be prepared to justify your actions to them.

## Relevant question – weaknesses
### What is your greatest weakness?

As this question often produces a 'stock answer', it is asked less and less frequently. However, when the question is asked there are some basic principles to adopt. Every individual has a weakness, and it would be foolish to suggest in an interview that you did not

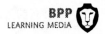

possess one. The panel is seeking proof of self-reflection, confirmation that the 'weakness' does not impact on patient safety, and that you have taken rectification steps. Commonly volunteered examples of weaknesses include: 'I'm not assertive enough', 'I often take work home', 'My time management skills are not ideal', 'My work/life balance is not great' and 'I do not delegate my responsibilities when maybe I should'. If you have taken obvious rectification steps, for instance the attendance and participation in a time management course, this information should be shared. These examples, though acceptable, serve as examples only. Be aware that if you give a stock response, this will exasperate the panel.

> *Relevant questions – investigating you further*
> 1. How do you deal with stress?
> 2. How do you cope with stress?
> 3. What are the major causes of stress to doctors?
> 4. How do you unwind after a hard day's work?
> 5. How do you ensure you maintain your work/life balance?
> 6. What are your hobbies? How do they influence your medical practice?

The working life of a doctor can place enormous stress on individuals which subsequently impacts on their colleagues and families. It is important to demonstrate to the interview panel that you are calm and collected, aware of the potential situations that can lead to stress and be able to manage it appropriately in the acute setting and also with a long-term strategy. The panel want to see doctors who lead a balanced working lifestyle.

There are some simple skills and steps that many develop in order to tackle stressful situations:

- The ability to step back and review the situation
- Identifying the key points causing the stress
- The ability to share concerns with colleagues
- Employing more effective time management tools
- Undertaking extra-curricular activities
- Ensuring you have regular holidays with those most important to you.

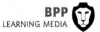

## Other general questions

1. Describe a difficult case and how you resolved it
2. I see from your CV that... Why did you do that?
3. What will you do if you do not get this job?
4. How do you keep up to date?
5. Are you a leader or a follower?
6. Do you think all doctors are leaders?
7. How many beds are in your Trust?
8. What tertiary services does your Trust provide?
9. Who is your Chief Executive/Medical Director? What is their background?
10. What job have you particularly liked/disliked?

The dreaded 'if you do not get this job' question, if asked at the start of the interview, will differentiate the pessimists from the optimists. The former may simply see this question as confirmation that they are not good candidates and will perform poorly in the rest of the interview. The optimists may simply see this question as a challenge and will demonstrate dedication to the panel.

Knowing the structure and key personnel in the Trust (where you are presently working at the time of the interview) will reassure the panel that you are an individual with an understanding of the importance of the infrastructure of an institution, and its impact on your working practices.

You can read a considerable amount of material to keep up-to-date both clinically and politically. Remember to include learned bodies, websites, journals, academic forums and newspapers. Regular journals or bulletins issued by Trusts may also be helpful in identifying key priorities and issues.

As mentioned briefly at the beginning of this chapter, the Consultant post has implicit and explicit needs for leadership. Historically, leadership has been thrust upon and expected from every doctor; unquestioning approaches to doctors' demands reinforced this. Unfortunately, this infrastructure has not lent itself in these modern questioning times, to the development of leadership skills for doctors who now find themselves having to rapidly develop the abilities they were historically expected to have.

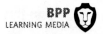

The need for development in this field is emphasised in the Tooke report (dealt with in later chapters), and further evidence for this is found in the numerous 'leadership' courses for medical staff and the 'Medical Leadership Competency Framework' (MLCF) from the Academy of Medical Royal Colleges.

The MLCF describes the leadership competencies doctors need in order to become more actively involved in the planning, delivery and transformation of health services. The Framework is a tool which can be used to:

- Inform the design of training curricula and development programmes
- Highlight individual strengths and development areas through self-assessment and structured feedback from colleagues
- Assist with personal development planning and career progression.

The Framework is well entrenched with the Academy of Medical Royal Colleges. They are continuing to work with the GMC to integrate the Framework into *Tomorrow's Doctors* and *Good Medical Practice*. The Postgraduate Medical Education and Training Board (PMETB) will integrate this into college curricula. The Framework applies to all medical students and doctors.

It would not be wise, therefore, to volunteer that 'I am always a follower'. However, it is clear that in addition to moments requiring genuine leadership, there are instances where it takes leadership qualities to follow. The latter is not an oxymoron, for example, you may be able to influence others to follow another person's lead.

'Management' duties may be encountered without too much difficulty during medical studentship and training. These duties may include:

- Warden duties in halls of residence
- President duties in the doctors' mess
- On call rota duties
- Delegated duties for:
    - Risk
    - Complaints
    - Audit

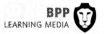

## Key points

- These questions aim to measure your self-awareness, standards, intellectual honesty, maturity and dependability
- Questions about the Post are designed to encourage the candidate to reflect on the benefits and drawbacks of the region, the Department, the clinical duties
- Questions about the Specialty may involve the identification of national or local challenges
- For questions on your qualities, avoid stock answers. Answers on self-description should give the panel an idea of the type of person you are; answers on ambition may relate to your career (specialty, Department, Trust) or personal issues. Remember the principles of being a good doctor
- For questions on your weaknesses, remember every individual has one. Demonstrate lack of impact on patient safety and rectification steps
- For questions on stress: demonstrate that you are calm and collected, aware of the potential situations that can lead to stress, and able to manage it appropriately
- Remind yourself of the ways you keep up-to-date
- Re-examine your leadership qualities and be aware of the MLCF
- Develop and reinforce your management duties
- Know the infrastructure of your present Trust

# Chapter 13

## Questions regarding scenarios

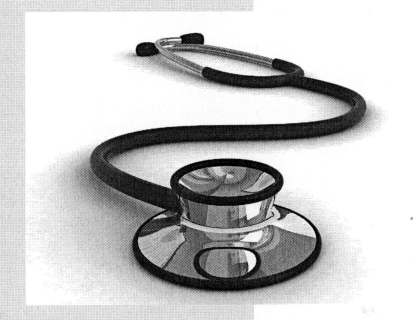

# Questions regarding scenarios

This has been briefly dealt with in a previous chapter; however scenario questions deserve special mention.

Scenario questions in the interview and psychometric assessments at stations test the candidate's methodology, wisdom, sharpness and decisiveness with regard to situations relating to key topics such as risk, complaints, fitness to practise, reputation (of the Department, the Trust, you and your colleagues), patient safety and welfare. As previously discussed, you should rapidly identify the issue or problem; this may be followed by a demonstration of your methodology with a short introductory explanation, for example 'I believe this is a question of professional/criminal conduct' or 'I believe this is a question of ethics'.

## *The specialty*

Imagine that the Deanery has asked you as a new Consultant to entertain some new Foundation doctors; you have been given one hour to describe your specialty to them. What would you discuss?

The aim of this question is to summarise the specialty succinctly, and highlight the attraction.

How would you dissuade a colleague from entering this specialty?

The disadvantages of the specialty are being sought. Clearly the candidate may wish to point out that in 'real life' there are several advantages which counterbalance the disadvantages.

Imagine that you have been successful in this interview, and we have transported you ten years into the future. What do you see?

This question deals with ambition, both for the individual and the Department/Trust.

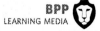

## Clinical risk

1. Could you talk us through all the stages that an adverse incident form goes through?
2. What could be the conclusion of a risk assessment for a needle stick injury?
3. What could be the conclusion of a risk assessment for the booking and performance of an investigation (eg blood test or X-ray) on the wrong patient?

The first question deals with the description of the risk process. The second and third questions deal with the process of education and dissemination of information.

Describe how you would deal with the situation if, a few months into your new Consultant post, you are called to a cardiac arrest in Accident and Emergency. The arrest is over, and the patient is dead. Your team inform you that this man had suffered an out-of-hospital cardiac arrest, and was found to have a shockable cardiac rhythm on arrival in Accident and Emergency. The defibrillator did not work, and a substitute was sought. By the time the substitute defibrillator was available, the situation was no longer salvageable. The family are waiting in the relatives' room.

This question deals with: empathy (the dissemination of information to the family); knowledge of the risk process (identifying the problem in the machine and the checking process, removing the machine from clinical circulation, and pursuing the submission and follow-up of the risk form); and time management (choosing the correct time to share information – it may be that the family require empathy there and then, while the machine incident may be discussed at a later date).

## Complaints

Describe how you would deal with the situation if four months into your new Consultant post, a patient verbally informs you of a grievance against:

1.  A staff nurse on your ward
2.  A junior doctor on your firm
3.  A Consultant colleague in your specialty

Awareness is needed of the procedures you may employ to: understand the patient and organise ways in which the issues may be dealt with, thereby minimising the chances of this grievance escalating.

Describe how you would deal with the situation if four months into your new Consultant post, a patient hands you a written complaint, describing grievances against:

1.  A Consultant colleague
2.  You and your team

This deals with your knowledge of the written complaints process. The strategies employed in the verbal complaint above may also be used to resolve the situation.

## Clinical effectiveness

Describe what you would do if, six months into your new Consultant post, you attend a very instructive clinical risk meeting which you feel would benefit patients through external scrutiny and openness.

The candidate is asked to describe the process of disseminating Trust information to the patients. The resources available should be described: directorate, clinical unit, operational manager, clinical director, Trust board, PALS, and the local media. Knowledge should be demonstrated that it is likely that the Trust will delegate this duty to an executive officer and PALS. The philosophy is that the dissemination of information should be seen as a constructive act by all parties.

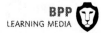

## Performance as a doctor

Describe how you would deal with the situation if a few months into your new Consultant post, you discover:

1. A Consultant colleague who appears to be: arriving late for work; leaving early from work; taking longer to make clinical decisions; the subject of some coffee room conversations about these issues
2. A Consultant colleague smelling of alcohol
3. A Consultant colleague appearing to be drunk at work
4. A Consultant colleague who is openly rude to patients and staff; this is noticed by patients
5. A senior Consultant colleague watching child pornography on his laptop in the coffee room
6. A junior doctor seemingly take a drug out of the drug cupboard, and put it in her mouth

The under-performing doctor requires empathy and assistance while the doctor performing unprofessionally or criminally requires going through due process. Patient safety is all important. Initially, it is vital that you confirm that any rumours or impressions are true, whether this applies to lateness, decision-making or smelling of alcohol. If the individual has not been unprofessional, a private discussion may be all that is required. It should be made clear that you will personally take an interest in the doctor's performance and that you may have no option other than discussing this further with your senior colleagues if necessary. Hopefully the under-performing doctor will appreciate these discussions; if however he/she refuses to enter into a discussion with you, you may have to rapidly organise a formal meeting with your senior colleagues.

If the issue with the doctor is a matter of fitness to practise (rudeness or criminal act), it is paramount that patients are protected. You should do your best to ensure that you discuss your intended actions with the doctor; the doctor is removed from the clinical scene (if appropriate); patient care is maintained with alternative clinical cover; you discuss this with the Clinical Director, medical director and the legal team; you follow up the Trust response to this individual; and you make further contributions to Trust decision making if you feel this is appropriate. It is also worth noting that

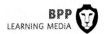

many criminal acts (such as watching child pornography) require immediate correspondence with the police; either you or the Trust can do this. It is also often appropriate that correspondence will be issued to the GMC on the grounds that there has been an issue of fitness to practise; this correspondence is often dealt with by the medical director.

> Describe how you would deal with the situation if a few months into your new Consultant post, you are offered:
>
> 1. Some money from a patient, in gratitude for your work
> 2. A bottle of wine from a patient's relative, in gratitude for your work
> 3. Some money for your department from a grateful patient

This question deals with an awareness of professional principles and probity. Money should never be accepted, unless a cheque is written to a nominated Trust charitable fund. Minor presents may be accepted at the discretion of the doctor. Gifts should be logged by all doctors, and letters of thanks should be issued by the Trust.

## Ethics and law

> Describe how you would deal with the situation if a few months into your new Consultant post:
>
> 1. An elderly gentleman on your ward has repeatedly seemingly withdrawn his consent to an intervention which may be life-saving
> 2. A patient has withdrawn her consent for an operation

The issues of consent have been dealt with in detail in a previous chapter. Knowledge of the principles of consent and an awareness of the Trust resources (such as psychiatry and the legal team) need to be demonstrated.

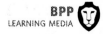

Describe how you would deal with the situation if a few months into your new Consultant post, your patient confidentially divulges his positive HIV status to you. He informs you that he is telling you this piece of information because he is worried that a new antibiotic drug that you have prescribed may react with some anti-retroviral drugs that he has been prescribed abroad. He does not want his GP, his wife or three other girlfriends to know his HIV status. He stresses that he simply requires reassurance regarding the drug reactions.

This question deals with empathy and consent. It would be prudent to explain to the patient that it is unlikely that drugs will interact, if this is the primary concern. Professional skills should be used to the maximum in order to convince that patient that sharing this information with health professionals and social contacts will lead to better clinical care for him and those around him. It is important that other healthcare professionals, who may have some experience in this field, are also involved. If after discussions the patient will not change his mind, he should be told that the Trust will inform external professionals in order for them to provide the best clinical care for the social contacts. Legal advice should be sought at all times.

Describe how you would deal with the situation if, a few months into your new Consultant post, you feel that ongoing treatment for a particular patient is futile.

1. How would you initiate the decision-making process?
2. Who would you involve in your discussions?
3. What are the responsibilities in the decision-making process of the patient, doctor, healthcare team, family members and other people who are close to the patient? What weight should be given to their views?

The de-escalation of treatment has been discussed elsewhere. The process should be multidisciplinary and multispecialty. The patient and relatives (the latter should be involved with the patient's consent, or in the event where the patient lacks capacity) should be intimately involved in discussions. There should be a clear distinction that relatives are not being burdened with the

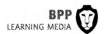

instruction to make a decision, but rather that their views will be closely listened to.

> A few months into your new Consultant post, an adverse incident on your ward comes to light. A drug with a risk of causing bleeding has been prescribed to the wrong patient. The risk form has been submitted. Describe how you would arrange to inform the patient, and what you would say.

Time should be taken to speak to the patient in private. Empathy should be used, and the language should be simple to understand. Reassurance should be given (if appropriate) that no harm has occurred and that the clinical situation will be closely monitored. A description to the patient of the error is important, together with any new processes which have been adopted for the prevention of a re-occurrence of this error. It is important that there should be a way for the patient to discuss any future queries with named healthcare professionals.

### Key points
You should:
- Be aware that scenario questions test the candidate's methodology, wisdom, sharpness and decisiveness with regard to situations relating to key topics
- Identify the topic being investigated
- Describe the process
- Be aware that patient safety is paramount and that professional standards must be upheld

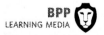

# Section 3

## History-related topics
### (Topics based on key points in history)

As mentioned elsewhere in this book, it is unlikely that you will be asked a random question on a key point. This is an interview, not an examination. However, knowledge of the political landscape will be important for your awareness of corporate anxieties and aspirations. A working (not exhaustive) knowledge of key points will allow you to provide coherent answers when asked of their relevance to your specialty.

# Chapter 14

## The Department of Health, and events up to the early 1990s

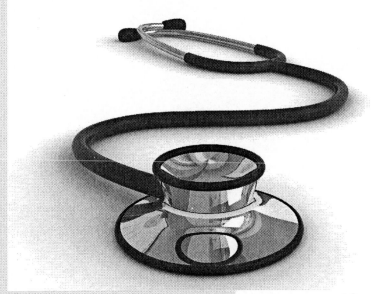

# The Department of Health, and events up to the early 1990s

## *The Department of Health*

The Department of Health (DoH) is a department of the United Kingdom government, responsible for policy on social care and public health, and is directly responsible for the National Health Service (NHS) in England. The English system is that which is described in detail in this chapter.

In other parts of the UK, responsibility for health and the management of the NHS has been devolved to local administrations:

- In Wales, the Welsh Assembly, strategic NHS Trusts and local Health Boards oversee healthcare
- In Scotland, the Scottish Executive Health Department and the NHS Boards wield the power. Clinical advice is given to these bodies by the Area Clinical Forum. Abolishment of NHS Trusts and PCTs occurred in 2004
- In Northern Ireland, the Northern Ireland Executive and the Health and Social Service Boards provide the central management system. In 2000, the project 'Investing for Health' was initiated (comparable in substance to the NHS Plan)

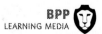

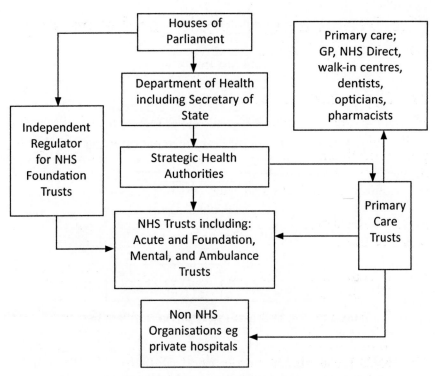

**Figure 14.1 The national structure of healthcare in England**

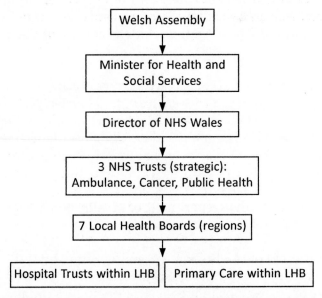

**Figure 14.2 The national structure of healthcare in Wales**

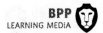

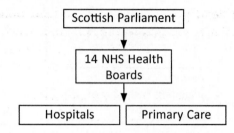

Figure 14.3 The healthcare structure in Scotland

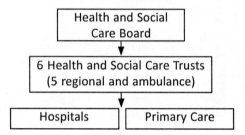

Figure 14.4 The healthcare structure in Northern Ireland

The DoH is led by the Secretary of State for Health, who is accountable to Parliament. Additional Ministers for Health report to the Health Secretary. They include the Minister of State for Health Services; Minister of State for Public Health; Parliamentary Undersecretary of State; Parliamentary Undersecretary for Health Services; and the Parliamentary Undersecretary of State for Care Services.

Some of the work of the DoH is carried out by 'arm's length bodies', including Executive Agencies such as NHS Estates, NHS Pensions Agency and the Medicines and Healthcare products Regulatory Agency (MHRA). Like many other UK state departments, the Department of Health has been known by various other names. It started out as the Board of Health, and then became known as the Ministry of Health. It was also for a time combined with social security (as the Department of Health and Social Security or DHSS, 1968–1988).

The Department of Health Board is an important body. It supports the Permanent Secretary, who is the Chair of the Board, in the discharge of his responsibilities as the Principal Accounting Officer for the Department.

There are three head policy advisors: the lead policy advisor on local government and social care, the head of finance and corporate functions, and three non-executive members who provide external input and challenge. The board is responsible for:

- Advice to ministers on developing the strategy and objectives for the health and social care system
- Setting DoH standards
- Establishing the framework of governance, assurance and management of risk
- Approving the:
  - Departmental Business Plan
  - Resource Accounts
  - Departmental Report
  - Major expenditure commitments as defined in scheme of delegations.

The DoH's Permanent Secretary is answerable to the Secretary of State and Parliament for the way the Department is run. As described above, he chairs the Department of Health Board, and therefore line manages the Social Care, Care Services, Equality and Human Rights, Communications, Corporate Management and Development directorates within the Department.

The NHS Chief Executive ensures that the Department provides strategic leadership for the NHS and social care.

The Chief Medical Officer (CMO) is the UK Government's principal medical adviser and leads key areas of the Department's work.

The other two executive directors are: the Director General of Social Care, Local Government and Care Partnerships and the Director General, Finance and Chief Operating Officer.

## Relevant question – the DoH

What do you think the DoH/Health Secretary/Chief Medical Officer's priorities are with regard to your specialty/this Trust?

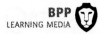

As in all factual questions, it is more likely that there will be relevance to topical or specialty-specific issues. As a general rule, the priorities for the DoH will be evident in:

- Your departmental managerial structure
- Medical journals
- Broadsheet newspapers
- Guidelines escalated to SHAs, PCTs and Chief Executives of acute trusts

## *The Griffiths Report (1983) – the introduction of general management*

In February 1983, the then Health Secretary Norman Fowler ordered an inquiry into the effective use of staffing and resources in the NHS. The report was led by Roy Griffiths, Deputy Chairman and Managing Director of Sainsbury's, in October 1983. He found that there was no coherent system of management at a local level. In addition, there seemed to be no evaluation of its performance against normal business criteria (quality, budgets, productivity, staff motivation, research and development). In June 1984 his recommendations were accepted by Parliament. Subsequently general managers were drawn from inside and outside the NHS in order to be introduced into health authorities and into hospitals and units by the end of 1985. Management budgets were introduced into hospitals as was the concept of 'value for money'.

The NHS Training Authority was established and programmes for management training and education were increased, particularly for doctors. It was considered essential that senior doctors in particular should be encouraged to become involved in the day-to-day management of the NHS. Various models were tried, though none was successful until the model of the 'clinical directorate' attracted support. This suggested that clinical services should be organised into a series of directorates which would each have a Clinical Director or lead Consultant, usually chosen by the other doctors within the directorate, to act on their behalf. The Clinical Director was expected to assume responsibility for providing leadership to the directorate and to represent the views of all the clinical specialties. He/she was expected to initiate change, agree workloads and resource allocation with the unit general manager,

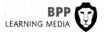

and act as the budget holder for the directorate. The relationship between the Clinical Director and colleagues was not seen as one of line management. Rather, the Clinical Director was expected to negotiate and persuade colleagues. Equally, the relationship between the Clinical Director and the unit general manager was seen as one of negotiation and persuasion.

The pace at which hospitals introduced clinical directorates varied widely. Eventually the philosophy evolved into the Clinical Director being 'in charge of the doctors' and the general manager remaining responsible for everyone else. The main drawback to implementing the Griffiths Report lay in the simple fact that the NHS had important differences from commercial businesses. There were no major incentives available to persuade those working in the NHS to change their ways of working. Furthermore, for poorly functioning hospitals, the traditional commercial sanctions of bankruptcy or takeovers could not apply; the hospital had to continue to offer a service.

## Relevant questions – the Directorate

1. What can you tell us about the Directorate management structure?
2. How does a Directorate improve its management style?
3. What does the future hold for doctors in management?

You may be able to demonstrate a working knowledge of the definition and history of the Directorate. In addition to referring to leadership issues (dealt with elsewhere in this book), it may be important to deal with the topics of quality, budgets, staff motivation and clinical governance.

## Working for patients (1989)

Heralded as the most formidable programme of reform in the history of the National Health Service in 1989, the DoH developed a White Paper in which plans were made for the creation of the internal market. These plans were the result of a year-long review of Health Services and were designed to make sure that the NHS was a service that put patients first. Efforts were also made to encourage and to organise medical audit within the internal

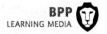

market. Protected funding for this was made available. The two main objectives were to:

1. Give patients better health care and greater choice of services
2. Provide greater satisfaction and rewards to NHS staff who successfully respond to local needs and preferences

The seven key measures were:

1. More delegation of responsibility to local level: in order to make the service more responsive to patients' needs, responsibilities were delegated from regions to districts and from districts to hospitals
2. Self-governing hospitals: to encourage a better service to patients, hospitals were able to apply for a new self-governing status within the National Health Service as NHS Hospital Trusts
3. New funding arrangements: hospitals which best met patients' needs should receive finances to do so; finances required to treat patients could cross administrative boundaries
4. Additional consultants: to reduce waiting times and improve the quality of service
5. GP Practice Budgets: to help the family doctor improve services for patients, large GP practices to be able to apply for their own NHS budgets to obtain a defined range of services direct from hospitals
6. Reformed management bodies: to improve the effectiveness of NHS management, regional, district and family practitioner management bodies to be reduced in size and reformed on business lines
7. Better audit arrangements: to ensure that all who deliver patient services make the best use of resources

Legislation was to be introduced at the earliest opportunity to give effect to those of the above proposals which required it.

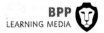

## The three phases

### Phase 1 (1989)

This was a year of preparation to identify the first self-governing hospitals. Regulations were introduced to facilitate easier changing of GP. The first additional Consultant posts were created.

### Phase 2 (1990)

The changes gathered momentum. 'Shadow' boards of the first self-governing hospitals (NHS Hospital Trust) started to develop plans for the future. Medical audit was extended.

### Phase 3 (1991)

The first NHS Hospital Trusts were established. The first GP practice budget holders began buying services. Health Authorities started paying directly for work they did for each other.

### Areas of concern at commencement:

- The White Paper concentrated on acute Health Services. There was a lack of Government plans for the development of community based and health provision for people with mental handicap and mental illness. There was no information on preventive health programmes, particularly those concerned with HIV, solvent abuse and alcoholism
- There were no specific plans for the co-ordination of community care services, for instance, close liaisons between Local Authorities and Health Authorities to ensure effective community care strategies
- Plans for large General Practices to run their own cash limited budgets, with scope to keep any money left over after they have bought treatment for their patients from hospitals and clinics were thought to discourage General Practitioners from taking on the elderly, the chronic sick and people who are disabled
- Plans were not made for patients treated in hospitals in another Health Authority's catchment area
- There was the risk that allowing hospitals to set their own priorities for any particular speciality they believed would bring in the most money would lead to a lack of incentives to provide expensive services which were seen as less profitable, eg the elderly

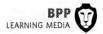

## *Relevant questions – the 'internal market'*

1. Do you believe in the 'internal market'?
2. How does the internal market affect your specialty?

The way to deal with 'opinion' questions has been dealt with elsewhere. The advantages and disadvantages should be identified and a pragmatic approach adopted. It is likely that there will be relevance to your specialty, as the internal market has widespread impact.

### Key points

- Regarding the Department of Health, you should know the basic relevance and history and be aware of new priorities which may have relevance to your specialty
- Be aware of the history of the introduction of management in the NHS
- Have a working knowledge of the definition and history of the Directorate
- Know the history and principles of the internal market, and their relevance to your specialty. Make sure you can refer to topics such as quality, budgets, staff motivation, research and development and audit
- Do not invest too much time in learning all the historical details. Rather, know the relevance of your specialty and its position with regard to the information above

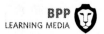

# Chapter 15

## The NHS Plan: precursors and consequences, including standards

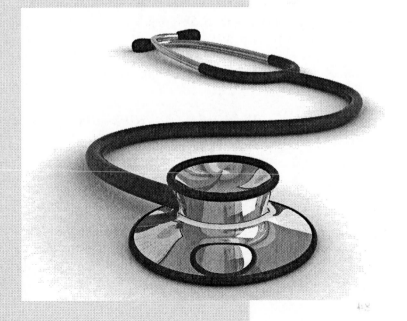

# The NHS Plan: precursors and consequences, including standards

## The New NHS (1997): modern and dependable

The Government set out its vision for the NHS in this White Paper published in December 1997. It described how the internal market would be replaced by a system called 'integrated care', based on partnership and driven by performance. It formed the basis for a ten-year programme to renew and improve the NHS through evolutionary change rather than organisational upheaval. These changes were designed to build on what had worked, but discard what had failed. The needs of patients were to be central to the new system.

However, by the winter of 1999/2000, hospitals were struggling and the NHS came under sustained attack for its failure to cope with winter pressures, the scarcity of intensive care beds, sub-standard cardiac and cancer care, and its uncaring treatment of elderly people. The Health Services Journal epitomised the NHS as 'under-funded, under pressure and under-appreciated'.

The Prime Minister at the time, Tony Blair, led the Government's reconsideration of its approach to the NHS. First, in March 2000, came a commitment to a substantial increase in funding for the NHS. Next came a period of work by specialist action teams and of consultation with NHS staff and the public to determine how to use this new money to best effect. The product was *The NHS Plan: A plan for investment, a plan for reform.*

## The NHS Plan: A plan for investment, a plan for reform (2000)

Despite its many achievements the NHS was seen to have failed to keep pace with changes in society. The NHS Plan outlined the vision of a health service designed around the patient. A new delivery system for the NHS together with changes between health and social services, changes for NHS doctors, for nurses, midwives, therapists and other NHS staff was proposed. There was also going to be a change in the relationship between the NHS and

 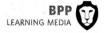

the private sector. The NHS Modernisation Board was set up to advise the Secretary of State for Health and his ministerial team on implementing The NHS Plan.

## *Ten core principles were established:*

1. A universal service for all based on clinical need, not ability to pay
2. A comprehensive range of services
3. Services shaped around the needs and preferences of individual patients, their families and carers
4. Responsiveness to the different needs of different populations
5. Continuous effort to improve quality services and minimise errors
6. The NHS to support and value its staff
7. Public funds for healthcare to be devoted solely to NHS patients
8. Working with others to ensure a seamless service for patients
9. Efforts to keep people healthy and reduce health inequalities
10. Respect for patient confidentiality, while providing open access to information about services, treatment and performance

## *'Public service agreement' targets:*

- A maximum wait of three months for outpatient appointments and six months for inpatient treatment by end 2005
- Two thirds of all outpatient appointments and inpatient elective admissions to be pre-booked by 2003/4, and 100 per cent by 2005
- Guaranteed access to a primary care professional within 24 hours, and to a primary care doctor within 48 hours, by 2004
- Year-on-year improvements in patient satisfaction
- To reduce the mortality rates substantially by 2010, of:
  - Heart disease (by at least 40 per cent in people under 75)
  - Cancer (by at least 20 per cent in people under 75)
  - Suicide and undetermined injury (by at least 20 per cent)

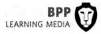

- To narrow the socio-economic and geographical health gap (specific targets to be developed in 2001)
- Trusts should meet value for money benchmarks for cost of care
- For the NHS to work in partnership with social services:
  - High quality pre-admission and rehabilitation care for older people
  - Year-on-year reductions in delay in moving people over 75 on from hospital
  - Increase the participation of problem drug-users in drug treatment programmes by 55 per cent by 2004, and 100 per cent by 2008

## Key financial features:

- Fixed 1999–2002 three-year settlement over-ridden by the March 2000 budget
- A commitment to an average annual NHS funding increase of 6.1 per cent UK in real terms over four years (2000–2004)
- Total NHS expenditure in England to rise from £44.5 billion (2000/1) to £56.7 billion (2003/4)
- A step change in capital investment to tackle long-term neglect
- Flexibility to carry over any unspent planned funding to the next year
- Increased resources

## Planned investments:

- Over 100 new hospitals between 2000 and 2010
- 7,000 extra beds in hospitals and intermediate care by 2004
- 1,700 extra non-residential intermediate care places
- 20 Diagnostic and Treatment Centres by 2004
- 500 new one-stop primary care centres, housing GPs, dentists, opticians, health visitors and social workers
- 250 new scanners, 45 new linear accelerators and other equipment
- Modern IT in NHS facilities, including patient access to electronic personal medical records and electronic prescribing by 2004
- Clean wards, better food, bedside televisions and telephones

- 7,500 more consultants and 2,000 more GPs by 2004
- 20,000 more nurses and over 6,500 more therapists by 2004
- Central funding for specialist registrar posts
- 1,000 more medical school places, in addition to 1,100 already announced, by 2005
- A new pay system for all NHS staff, and extra pay in shortage areas
- Childcare support, including 100 subsidised, on-site nurseries by 2004
- Improvements in occupational health and the working environment
- £140 million more for staff development, and a Leadership Centre.

## Changes to staff:

- All NHS doctors were to participate in annual appraisal and clinical audit, including rapid mechanisms for handling under-performance and poor performance, including a new National Clinical Assessment Authority
- The majority of GPs were to join the Personal Medical Services scheme by 2004; a revised, quality-based national contract existed for the remainder
- The option was available for GPs to work on a full-time or part-time salaried basis
- Hospital care was to become Consultant-delivered. This was dependent on a new Consultant contract, which involved mandatory appraisal, effective job plans and approximately seven fixed sessions per week. There was scope for additional remuneration through accreditation. There was a suggestion that new consultants were to work exclusively for the NHS for 'perhaps' their first seven years; during this time they would provide perhaps eight fixed sessions per week, together with an increased amount of out of hours service
- New skills and roles were to be given to nurses, midwives and therapists; these would include running clinics, ordering diagnostic tests, prescribing drugs etc
- 1,000 nurse consultants by 2004, and new consultant therapists
- Modern matrons with clear authority on the wards
- Strengthened regulation of the clinical professions

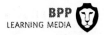

## *Changed systems:*

- Streamlining occurred at the top of the DoH; a single, more autonomous Chief Executive was responsible for public health functions, the NHS and social services, and reported to a new NHS Modernisation Board on delivery of the NHS Plan
- 'Earned autonomy' was planned for NHS organisations
- Core national standards and targets were agreed
- A Modernisation Agency was developed to support best practice and improvement
- A mandatory reporting system for adverse healthcare events was devised
- Independent inspection by the Commission for Health Improvement (CHI) was planned
- It was agreed that there should be independent publication of performance information
- £500 million Performance Fund was set up to reward good performance, and intervention was arranged in the case of poor performance
- Local government was asked to scrutinise the NHS locally

## *Inequality targets:*

- Public Service Agreement (PSA) national health inequalities targets should be scrutinised
- By 2002 a new health poverty index was to be set up to combine data about health status, access to health services, uptake of preventive services, and opportunities to maintain health
- Reducing inequalities should become a key criterion for NHS resource allocation by 2003
- The NHS Performance Framework Action was to assess actions to reduce inequalities
- New formulae and incentives were designed to improve the distribution of primary care staff; Medical Practices Committee was abolished
- New screening programmes to be instituted
- Free fruit to be made available for young school children

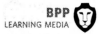

## *Patient convenience:*

- NHS Direct was to become a one-stop gateway to out-of-hours healthcare by 2004
- Better out-of-hours pharmacy services were to be developed: more over-the-counter medicines, repeat prescriptions from the pharmacist, and delivery of medicines to the patient's door
- More tests and treatment in primary care (as opposed to hospital consultants) and up to 1,000 new specialist GPs
- On-the-spot booking systems to be created for hospital appointments
- NHS Direct nurses were to check on older people living alone
- Free translation and interpretation services to be provided in all NHS premises via NHS Direct

## *Older people:*

- A National Care Standards Commission to be set up in 2002 to drive up standards in domiciliary and residential care
- A National Service Framework on services for older people was to commence
- Resuscitation policies would be a requirement in all NHS organisations
- A pilot was to start in 2001 of a free NHS retirement health check
- Breast screening would be provided for women aged 65–70
- Personal care plans would exist for all
- There would be a new 'Care Direct' service, giving more home care and support as well as more intermediate care
- Subject to Parliament, there would be free nursing care in nursing homes (but not free personal care)

## *Patient information and empowerment:*

- A Patient Advocacy and Liaison Service (PALS) was to exist in every Trust by 2002
- There would be a reform of procedures for complaints and 'informed consent'
- A new NHS Charter would be developed by 2001

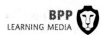

- The abolition of Community Health Councils would occur, in favour of a Patients' Forum in every Trust and a local advisory forum in every Health Authority
- There would be patient and/or citizen representation on the NHS Modernisation Board, and every Trust Board and CHI team(s)
- A new Independent Reconfiguration Panel was to advise on contested major service changes
- A new Citizens' Council would advise NICE on clinical assessment.

## Performance targets:

- The NHS Plan (2000) proposed that NHS organisations should be performance-assessed against government targets and priorities (set out in the Plan) and given ratings
- These ratings were published by the Department of Health for the first time in September 2001, in respect of acute hospital Trusts only (based on their performance in 2000–1)
- All acute Trusts in England were rated on their performance against Key targets (using the rating options for each target of 'achieved', 'underachieved' and 'significantly under-achieved'). They were also rated (using a five-point scale) on the following focus areas:
  - Clinical focus
  - Patient focus
  - Capacity and capability
- Trusts were assessed using a 'balanced scorecard' method (intended to allow for the relative strengths and weaknesses of each individual organisation) to produce an overall composite assessment from zero to three stars
- In July 2002 acute Trusts received their second annual ratings (relating to performance in 2001–2) alongside the first performance ratings for specialist hospital Trusts and ambulance Trusts (using the same system for acute Trusts). The performance of Primary Care Organisations was assessed for the first time against a range of suitable indicators, but they were not given an overall star rating

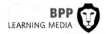

## The Commission for Health Improvement (CHI) (1997)

In December 1997, the idea for a commission for health improvement was mooted in New Labour's first health policy White Paper, *The New NHS*. It proposed an arm's length statutory body to 'monitor, assure and improve' clinical systems in NHS providers, with powers to intervene in failing trusts. In June 1998, yet another White Paper, *A First Class Service – Quality in the NHS*, was published, outlining further details of how CHI would work and including its role as a 'trouble-shooter'. By June 1999, the Health Act (1999) received royal assent and the CHI was created. Operations began in April 2000, and publications of the first routine clinical governance reviews were completed in December 2000.

August 2001 presented another landmark, when Epsom and St Helier Hospitals NHS Trust was the subject of the CHI's critical routine inspection report. It uncovered high death rates, 20-hour trolley waits, filthy toilets and patient complaints that took too long to resolve. The Trust Chief Executive became the first manager to resign directly as a result of a CHI report. In November 2001 the NHS reform bill was published. This followed the recommendations of the July 2001 public inquiry into children's heart surgery at Bristol Royal Infirmary. The bill proposed new powers for an NHS inspectorate, including the ability to suspend services at failing trusts, to inspect private health facilities where NHS work was carried out and to publish an annual state-of-the-NHS report. In response to this the Chancellor at the time, Gordon Brown, made a budget speech in April 2002, outlining a five-year 43 per cent increase in NHS funding. He unveiled plans for a new super-inspectorate to keep track of NHS performance. Subsequently, the NHS Reform Act 2002 expanded the powers of CHI to include performance assessment of the NHS. This indicated that CHI would publish NHS star ratings in future. The performance ratings published by CHI in July 2003 (relating to 2002–3) covered all acute, specialist, ambulance and mental health Trusts, and all Primary Care Trusts (PCTs).

Subsequently, CHI was merged with the Mental Health Act Commission, the National Care Standards Commission and parts of the Audit Commission to form the Commission for Healthcare Audit and Inspection (CHAI), which became operational from April

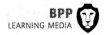

2004 (a new Commission for Social Care Inspection for England was also created at the same time). It was subsequently decided that CHAI would be known as the Healthcare Commission (HCC).

## The Healthcare Commission (HCC) (2004)

The Healthcare Commission (HCC) was established under the Health and Social Care (Community Health and Standards) Act 2003 and was known in legislation by its full name, the Commission for Healthcare Audit and Inspection. The Commission came into being on 1 April 2004 and had the general function of encouraging improvement in the provision of health care by and for NHS bodies in England and Wales. The Commission's functions included:

- The work previously undertaken by CHI (the latter ceased to exist in March 2004)
- The private and voluntary healthcare work of the National Care Standards Commission (NCSC); this also ceased to exist in March 2004. The NCSC was an independent body established by the Care Standards Act 2000, responsible for regulating independent sector care services, including healthcare services, in England
- The work of the Audit Commission, relating to value for money in healthcare. The Audit Commission is an independent organisation that promotes the best use of public money by local authorities and other bodies – it has additional powers under best value legislation

The HCC powers therefore covered two distinct though complementary roles – audit and inspection. The Commission was also given a range of new functions including handling the second stage of the NHS complaints process and the co-ordination of reviews into healthcare. The Commission published its new Annual Health Check in October 2006 which provided in-depth performance measurements of NHS trusts.

The Quality of Services score was an aggregation of each Trust's scores when assessed against the following benchmarks, set by the government:

- Core Standards. In respect of each individual core standard, Trusts were rated using the options 'compliant', 'insufficient assurance' or 'not met'. This lead to an overall rating of 'fully met', 'almost met', 'partly met' or 'not met'
- Existing National Targets (using the rating options 'fully met', 'almost met', 'partly met' or 'not met')
- New National Targets (using the rating options 'excellent', 'good', 'fair' or 'weak')

If an organisation scored 'not met' for either Core Standards or Existing National Targets, it was automatically given a score of 'weak' for Quality of Services. This was the only way that an organisation could receive a score of 'weak' for Quality of Services. Different rules applied to mental health Trusts.

## *The Care Quality Commission (2008)*

Since 2008 a single regulatory body for health and social care was created by the government by merging the HCC with the Commission for Social Care Inspection and the Mental Health Act Commission. This formed the Care Quality Commission (CQC).

Overall, Quality of Services scores are still not directly comparable across different organisation types (PCTs, acute Trusts, Ambulance Trusts, etc). This is a result of the differing number of Existing Targets and New National Targets that apply to each type. Direct comparisons of overall Quality of Services scores are thus only valid within an individual organisation type (ie when comparing PCTs with PCTs, acute Trusts with acute Trusts, etc).

In each annual assessment, Trusts are still required to assess themselves and submit declarations on how far they have achieved each Core Standard, using sets of criteria issued by the CQC. As part of the declaration process, Trusts are responsible for seeking commentaries on their performance against Core Standards from 'third parties'. These may be Strategic Health Authorities, Patient and Public Involvement Forums (Local Involvement Networks from 2008–9), Local Authority Health Overview and Scrutiny Committees or Elected Governors (in the case of Foundation Trusts). Third parties are not expected to sign off or directly comment on Trusts' declarations. Rather, the Trusts must include

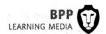

third-party commentaries, word-for-word, with their declarations. In turn, the third party commentaries are cross-checked against Trusts' declarations. Depending on the information received from third parties, the Trust may be investigated further, by means of a risk-based inspection (to which around 10 per cent of Trusts are subjected each year).

Random inspections are also carried out for the purpose of quality assurance (involving a further 10 per cent of Trusts each year). According to its findings, penalty points may be deducted and Trusts' declarations may be adjusted, where appropriate.

The significant changes to the annual assessments performed by the CQC as opposed to the HCC included the following:

- All acute Trusts are now inspected to check on compliance with the Hygiene Code
- PCTs are assessed on their performance as commissioners of services, separately from their performance as service providers
- Assessment against 'National Priorities' have replaced the measurement of performance against 'Existing National Targets' and 'New National Targets'

You should be aware of the high profile national targets set by the government year-upon-year. Many or all of these will have some bearing on your specialty.

## Relevant questions – the NHS Plan

1. Where have we got to regarding the NHS Plan and your specialty?
2. Has the NHS Plan delivered for your specialty?
3. What exposure have you had to the CQC?
4. How are standards measured for your specialty/the Trust?
5. Are you aware of the interfaces your specialty has with the CQC?
6. In what ways do you think your specialty can maintain/ improve this Trust's standards, as measured by external bodies?

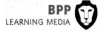

- What processes could you help put in place to set standards for your specialty?
- What do you think is the most significant government target with regard to your specialty?
- What is the most recent significant government target with regard to your specialty?

The CQC and the maintenance of Government standards are topics which form the basis for many sleepless nights for Chief Executives and Medical Directors! Status for excellence (and indeed Foundation status) will depend on the success or failure in achieving these standards. It is understandable, therefore, that these issues will be revisited time and time again in various Trust forums. It follows that a solid understanding of the relevance of Government standards to your specialty, and ideas for pursuing these standards, will play a fundamental role in the outcome of the interview. After dealing with Government standards, you must not forget to mention the standards pertaining to quality and academia.

### Key points

- Be aware of the relevance of The NHS Plan, its key principles and its relevance
- Be aware of the historical development of the Care Quality Commission (CQC) and its precursors
- Do not invest too much time in learning all the historical details. Rather, know the relevance of your specialty and its position with regard to the NHS plan, and your specialty's interface with the CQC, standards and targets

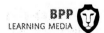

# Chapter 16

## Other bodies and philosophies which evolved from the NHS Plan

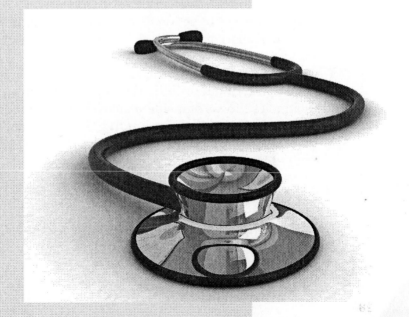

# Other bodies and philosophies which evolved from the NHS Plan

## *Adverse healthcare events and risk*

An expert report on risk in the NHS (*An organisation with a memory*) was conducted by the Department of Health in 2000, led by the Chief Medical Officer. It was found that the adverse incidents, though uncommon, had devastating consequences. The consequences were costly, and there was a familiar ring to most of the errors. The problems at the outset were:

- Often the picture was incomplete
- 400 people died or were seriously injured in adverse events involving medical devices
- Nearly 10,000 people were reported to have experienced serious adverse reactions to drugs
- Around 1,150 people with recent contact with mental health services committed suicide
- Nearly 28,000 written complaints were made about aspects of clinical treatment in hospitals
- The NHS paid out around £400 million a year settlement of clinical negligence claims
- There was an estimated liability of around £2.4 billion for existing and expected claims
- Hospital-acquired infections – around 15 per cent of which may have been avoidable – were estimated to have cost the NHS nearly £1 billion
- The NHS was not good at learning lessons: when things went wrong an individual or individuals were identified to carry the blame. The focus of incident analysis had tended to be on the events immediately surrounding an adverse event, and in particular on the human acts or omissions immediately preceding the event itself.

The proposed way forward:

- Unified mechanisms were recommended for reporting, and analysis when things go wrong
- A more open culture

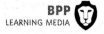

- Mechanisms for ensuring that the necessary changes were put into practice
- A much wider appreciation of the value of the system approach in preventing, analysing and learning from errors

In the following year (2001) a further report (*Adverse healthcare events: Building a Safer NHS for Patients*) was issued by the Department of Health. The Government accepted all the recommendations in *An organisation with a memory*, and also accepted that successful implementation depended on:

- The commitment of all NHS staff and the boards of all NHS organisations and Trusts
- The creation of a culture where staff feel that they can report errors, mistakes and adverse events without fear of retribution
- The establishment of clear national and local mechanisms for reporting mistakes and near misses and analysing trends
- The learning of lessons to reduce risk and prevent future harm to patient

Outcomes from the reports described above:

- The National Patient Safety Agency (NPSA), established in July 2001, co-ordinates efforts to identify and learn from mistakes. Health workers are encouraged to report incidents that they have witnessed without fear of reprimand. The NPSA is looking at how the public could report to it directly using the internet or a confidential hotline
- The Clinical Negligence Scheme for Trusts had already existed since 1994. It was essentially an insurance mechanism which Trusts use to fund the costs of litigation and provide effective management of claims. It is administered by the NHS Litigation Authority (NHSLA). NHSLA as the provider of cover, visits Trusts regularly to ensure that patient safety-related issues (for instance maternity and midwife processes, clinical equipment) are of a sufficient standard. The grading of the patient safety profile standard issued by NHSLA to the Trust relates to the amount of money a Trust pays for cover. The topics on the agenda for the NHSLA visits will vary from time to time

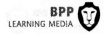

- The National Reporting and Learning System (NRLS) draws together reports of patient safety incidents and systems failures from health professionals across England and Wales. It helps the NHS to understand the underlying causes of problems and act quickly to introduce practical change
- An integrated approach to investigating errors across the NHS and different agencies
- The following authorities developed relationships to the bodies above:
  - The National Clinical Assessment Authority (a special health authority set up to provide a support service to health authorities and hospital and community trusts faced with concerns over the performance of an individual doctor. It is now part of the NPSA as the 'National Clinical Assessment Service, NCAS')
  - The General Medical Council (GMC)
  - The Care Quality Commission (CQC)

## Relevant questions – clinical risk

1. Have you had any dealings with your Trust's Risk Department? How does it work?
2. How many types of meetings have you attended recently, which have dealt with clinical risk?
3. Can you recall being involved in a clinical situation which involved clinical risk? How was it dealt with?
4. How is risk dealt with in your present department or directorate?
5. Have you ever filled in a 'Serious untoward incident' (SUI) form? Whose hands did it go through? What actions did you take to follow up?
6. Has your department any strong interfaces with the NPSA/ NRLS?

It is probable that most days in clinical practice involve decisions about or assessment of clinical risk. Ideally most NHS directorates and departments should have specific meetings for risk, which all doctors should regularly attend. Sadly, this is not the case at present. It is important therefore that doctors, particularly senior trainees, identify risk meetings relevant to their specialty, and make a point of regularly attending. All Trusts and all directorates have

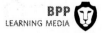

registers of clinical and non-clinical risk. There should be evidence of consistent handling and cross-directorate learning.

It is vital that any 'adverse incident' forms are followed through. A thorough understanding is essential of: the type of personnel in the department responsible for risk; their responsibilities in dealing with adverse incidents; the process of actions; method of recommendations. It is good practice for the individuals responsible for submission of the adverse incident form to check the status of assessment. Conversely, the risk department should as a matter of course feedback to these individuals.

## NHS Direct

This is a 24-hour, confidential telephone, online and interactive digital TV health advice and information service provided by the National Health Service in England and Wales. The organisation has been given Special Health Authority status. It was rolled out between 1998 and 2000, and a similar service was introduced in Scotland in 2004 (where it is called NHS24). The telephone service aims to triage callers to provide guidance on which healthcare provider the caller should access. Nurses also give advice on how to manage an episode of illness at home. In some areas of the UK, NHS Direct is commissioned by local Primary Care Trusts to provide the gateway for out-of-hours access to GP's surgeries and clinics, and also to emergency and routine NHS dentistry. The website contains a self-help guide and also a comprehensive health encyclopaedia. There is also an online enquiry service, which is similar to the telephone-based health information service, where visitors to the site can request information via email.

## National Service Frameworks

These are long term strategies for improving specific areas of care, such as UK's largest causes of morbidity and mortality, other common conditions and key patient groups. They set national standards, identify key interventions and put in place agreed time scales for implementation. These aims are achieved by being inclusive – developed in partnership with health professionals, patients, carers, health service managers, voluntary agencies and other experts. The topics at present are:

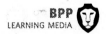

- Cancer
- Mental health
- Children
- Chronic obstructive pulmonary disease (COPD)
- Coronary artery disease
- Diabetes
- Long-term conditions (neurological and other)
- Stroke
- The elderly

Two main roles include:

1. The setting of clear quality requirements for care based on the best available evidence of what treatments and services work most effectively for patients
2. The offering of strategies and support to help organisations achieve these

## Relevant questions – NSF standards

1. What examples of NSF standards can you give me for your specialty?
2. How would you maintain these standards?

These questions investigate the same issues as those dealing with standards relating to the CQC.

## The Patient Advocacy and Liaison Service (PALS)

The NHS Plan set out to establish a new system of patient and public involvement (PPI) to replace Community Health Councils in England as part of the modernisation programme. The system was also designed to respond to the Bristol Royal Inquiry report, which recommended representation of patient interests 'on the inside' of the NHS and at every level. PALS are available in all Trusts and are a central part of PPI in England. They provide:

- Confidential advice and support to patients, families and their carers
- Information on the NHS and health related matters

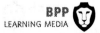

- Confidential assistance in resolving problems and concerns quickly
- Information on and explanations of NHS complaints procedures and how to get in touch with someone who can help
- Information on how you can get more involved in your own healthcare and the NHS locally
- A focal point for feedback from patients to inform service developments
- An early warning system for NHS Trusts, Primary Care Trusts and Patient and Public Involvement Forums by monitoring trends and gaps in services and reporting these to the trust management for action
- Liaisons with staff, managers and, where appropriate, other relevant organisations, to negotiate speedy solutions and to help bring about changes to the way that services are delivered
- Referrals for patients and families to local or national-based support agencies, as appropriate

## Relevant questions – PALS

1. Have you had any dealings with PALS?
2. Have you ever witnessed a complaint from a patient or a relative about you, your colleagues or your department? What was the outcome?
3. Are you aware of what 'PALS' do (other than deal with complaints)?

## Data

The Data Protection Act in 1984 ensured that any data possessed would be relevant, accurate, updated and processed formally. It was not to be disclosed, and kept only as long as necessary. Individuals (ie patients, their representatives and staff) had right to access and amendment and guaranteed security.

The following safeguards were implemented for healthcare institutions:

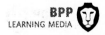

- There should be a named guardian or custodian to ensure confidentiality (referred to as 'Caldicott Guardians', after Dame Fiona Caldicott)
- There should be strict terms of internet usage
- There should be standardised application of security including methods of storage and generation of passwords

Joint guidance was produced by the BMA and NHS Connecting for Health:

- Everyone in the NHS has a responsibility to understand the implications of dealing with electronic patient data
- NHS Code of Confidentiality
- Always log-out of any computer system or application when work on it is finished and do not leave a terminal unattended and logged-in
- Do not share logins with other people and do not reveal passwords to others
- Change passwords at regular intervals and avoid using obvious passwords
- Always clear the screen of a previous patient's information before seeing another
- Use a password-protected screen-saver to prevent casual viewing of patient information by others

Organisational responsibilities:

- Each organisation should have security, information governance and records management policies in place, which should be *endorsed by the Board* or senior partners and updated at regular intervals
- The default position is there should be no transfers of unencrypted person identifiable data held in electronic format across the NHS
- Organisations must ensure that staff are aware of good practice with regard to security
- Each staff member should receive regular training

At the time of writing, there is no obvious commitment to a huge national project for the handling of data – this is particularly relevant as there had over the last decade been a history of bad

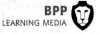

management. Local and regional projects are likely to be key. There will be strong interfaces with European Work Time Directive and Modernising Medical Careers; with the shortened day and career span of the trainee doctor, data handling should be efficient to enable the doctor to return to the bedside. Clearly, data models should also map to the needs of institutions and clinicians for meeting quality and other targets.

## *Choose and Book (CaB)*

Introduced from 2005 onwards, this application enables patients needing an outpatient appointment to choose which hospital they are referred to by their general practitioner, and to book a convenient date and time for their appointment. It was procured as part of the National Project for Information Technology (NPfIT) in 2003. Surgery where immediate treatment is required is not in the remit of Choose and Book. Such patients' needs bypass any longer-term queuing systems. In its fully functional mode, Choose and Book communicates electronically between 'compliant' GP Clinical Computer systems and Hospital Patient Administration Systems (PAS). For a number of reasons several GP and PAS Systems have not been made compliant in time to deliver the Choose and Book targets set by the Department of Health. Interim solutions were devised to allow patients to benefit from CaB during 2005/6.

Web-based Referral (WBR) allows a GP to access Choose and Book via a standard web browser until their Clinical Computing system can be successfully upgraded.

Indirectly Bookable Services (IBS) enables telephone call handlers in hospitals to offer CaB appointments to patients.

The commencement of CaB in 2005 suffered some delays: some technical (as a result of its dependency on other NPfIT work streams), some functional (problems in early releases), and some through clinicians' concerns about additional workloads. However, since the application became more stable during 2005, volumes have increased steadily. Where it is being used most patients report an improved service and like it. However, there have been detractors who have been put off by the idea of booking online. Some patients have complained that the system is too confusing. In addition, it is still possible to book through CaB without entering some important

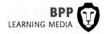

clinical data, and there are anecdotal reports that much relevant information pertaining to the nature of the referral/booking is lost when viewed at the provider end. For example, it has been documented on occasions that doctors seeing CaB patients in the Outpatient Department do not have any information other than the name of the patients and demographics.

## Relevant questions – CaB

1. Do you have electronic patient records where you work?
2. What are the benefits and drawbacks?
3. How could information technology impact better with your specialty?
4. What are the controversies these days in information technology?
5. Are you in favour of Choose and Book?
6. Does Choose and Book work?

## The National Institute for Health and Clinical Excellence (NICE)

The National Institute for Health and Clinical Excellence (NICE) is a Special Health Authority of the National Health Service. It commenced as the 'National Institute for Clinical Excellence' in 1999, and in April 2005 amalgamated with the Health Development Agency to become the 'National Institute for Health and Clinical Excellence' (still abbreviated as NICE). It was originally established to review clinical approaches, and also help defuse the so-called 'postcode lottery' system of healthcare, where the application of some effective therapies at times seemingly depended upon where patients happened to live. NICE publishes appraisals of particular treatments, and provides recommendations upon their effectiveness, and cost- effectiveness. NICE assessments must take into account both desired medical outcomes and also economic arguments regarding differing treatments.

Since 2005, the NHS in England and Wales has been legally obliged to provide funding for medicines and treatments recommended by NICE. The appraisal of an intervention or technology by NICE goes through discrete stages:

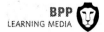

- The intervention or technology must have been referred to NICE by the Secretary of State for Health
- The ensuing appraisal stage includes patient groups, organisations representing health care professionals and the manufacturers of the product undergoing appraisal. Also, additional organisations are included, such as manufacturers of products to which the product undergoing appraisal is being compared
- An independent academic centre then draws together and analyses all of the published information on the technology under appraisal and prepares an assessment report
- Comments are then taken into account and changes made to the assessment report to produce an evaluation report
- An independent Appraisal Committee then looks at the evaluation report, and hears spoken testimony from clinical experts, patient groups and carers. They take their testimony appraisal consultation document
- This is sent to all consultees and commentators who are then able to make further comments
- Once these comments have been taken into account the final document is drawn up. This is called the final appraisal determination
- This is submitted to NICE for approval

At the time of writing, although it is not mandatory for Trusts to follow NICE guidelines, it is nevertheless mandatory for the Trust to report its actions with regard to new NICE guidelines. NICE is but one credible source, sometimes in a selection of many. On occasions, guidelines from different credible sources may conflict. It is up to professionals to demonstrate that guidelines pertaining to their specialty have been discussed in appropriate forums, and the reasoning for adopting certain policies is documented.

The mandatory reportable issues for NICE guidelines are:

- Is the new guideline relevant to your Trust? (ie is the activity described in the guideline performed at all? If not, there are no further questions to answer)
- If the guideline is relevant, is it appropriate? (ie is the guideline implemented fully/partially/not at all?)

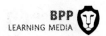

- If not fully, why not? (Here, a systematic response is required; it is not acceptable to say 'the guideline is rubbish' or 'we just do not agree'. Rather, acceptable responses may include the lack of modernisation of the NICE guideline when measured against best available evidence and consequent preference for an alternative guideline)

Whether you accept the arguments of NICE acceptance by clinicians or not, it should be recognised that commissioners may steer (rightly or wrongly) towards Trusts which *do* utilise NICE guidelines, and patients may do the same. It is implicit therefore that there may be a credibility issue linked to NICE acceptance and financial penalties (commissioners' choices) with NICE rejection.

## Relevant questions – NICE

1. What is the role of NICE?
2. Tell us about the two most recent NICE guidelines relating to your specialty. Did you and your department adopt them? Why/why not?
3. Should we always adopt NICE guidelines?

## Acute Trusts

Acute Trusts run hospitals (see the recent chapter on the 'NHS Plan'). Unless they are Foundation Trusts, they are accountable to the Strategic Health Authority. There are, in addition, Mental Health Trusts, Ambulance Trusts and Children's Trusts (which include health, education, social services).

## Foundation Trusts

NHS Foundation Trusts (often referred to as 'Foundation Hospitals') are hospitals which are non-profit making, are part of the NHS and have a similar relationship with PCTs to non-Foundation Trusts. Nevertheless, they have a significant amount of managerial and financial freedom which non-Foundation Trusts do not have. The introduction of NHS Foundation Trusts represented a profound change in the history of the NHS and the way in which hospital services were managed and provided. The philosophy centres on 'ownership' by the local community and therefore a 'patient-led'

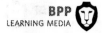

NHS. This is achieved (or attempted to be achieved) by more significant representation of the community on the Board of Governors. The original purpose was to devolve decision-making from a centralised NHS to local communities; the cynics saw the change towards semi-independent hospital boards as a move towards privatisation of the health service.

A key difference for foundation trusts is that they are not accountable to the local Strategic Health Authority, but rather directly to the Department of Health through the Independent Regulator ('Monitor'). Technically, they are not even under the directorship of the Secretary of State. The first ten such Trusts were approved in April 2004.

| Advantages of Foundation Trusts | Perceived disadvantages/limitations of Foundation Trusts |
|---|---|
| Faster decision making in financial matters are possible | A restriction is placed on the number of private patients which can be treated |
| There is more flexibility in financial matters (eg borrowing) | If there is a conflict in philosophies in service provision between the Board of Governors/community and the PCT, the wishes of the PCT may still carry greater influence (as a result of contractual obligations) than the wishes of the Board of Governors. It is more prevalent to find common ground, though |
| There is more opportunity to plan ahead strategically | |
| In theory, there is greater community influence in the running of the Trust by way of the community representation in the Board of Governors | |

## Relevant questions (if you are applying to a Foundation Trust or a Trust applying for Foundation status)

1. What are the advantages or disadvantages of Foundation Trusts?
2. Would our status as Foundation Trust make us more or less attractive to you? Why?
3. How could your specialty help us succeed in becoming a Foundation Trust?

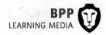

Yet again, this last question is related to standards and Healthcare Commission pressures, as successful applications for Foundation status are based on sound financial plans and clinical standards.

## *Primary Care Trusts*

All primary care services are managed by local Primary Care Trusts (PCTs). They exist to service local NHS needs and to ensure satisfactory numbers and quality of General Practitioners. In addition to these management responsibilities, Primary Care Trusts also commission the provision of the care provided by NHS Hospital Trusts.

PCTs also work with Local Authorities and other agencies that provide health and social care locally to make sure that local community's needs are being met. Primary Care Trusts are now at the centre of the NHS and receive 75 per cent of the NHS budget. As they are local organisations, they are in the best position to understand the needs of their community, so they can make sure that the organisations providing health and social care services are working effectively.

Individual/group practices may hold and manage an indicative budget for health care. This is called 'practice-based commissioning'. The savings are used to improve local services (with PCT approval). Legally the PCTs still hold the budgets, and the risks, and are responsible for delivery of targets.

The 'lead PCT' hosts and manages the allocated budget for the SHA area. It also handles disputes between constituent PCTs, and provides expertise on local procurement issues. It may lead on the prioritisation of investment proposals. At times the lead PCT may be a virtual arrangement, rather than a physical one.

The Department of Health calculates a 'target allocation' for every PCT based on four key factors:

- Numbers
- Need
- Distance from target
- Pace of change

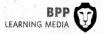

## Relevant questions – PCTs

1. How do you think PCTs see your specialty?
2. How do you think partnerships between acute Trusts and PCTs could be developed in your specialty? If we were to appoint you, how could you develop our relationship/partnership with the PCT?

There is a drive for acute Trusts to work more in partnership with PCTs. This is a consequence of the Darzi report (see Chapter 27) and the 'patient-led NHS' . There may in addition, be finances available for relevant treatment directly in the gift of the PCT, whereas the Trust may have more pressing financial pressures. Although informal 'networking' occurs between Consultants and GPs, ideas for innovations for working in partnership with PCTs should be formally examined by the Trust Board. Ideas from Consultants, therefore, should be discussed with the Chief Executive, who may then organise meetings within the Trust to facilitate liaisons with the PCT.

## Strategic Health Authorities

These were created by the Government in 2002 to manage the local NHS on behalf of the Secretary of State. In particular, they were to ensure robust Lead PCT arrangements were in place, and that investments in capital schemes reflected national and local strategic priorities. There were originally 28. In July 2006, this number was reduced to 10. Fewer, more strategic organisations were thought to be able to oversee stronger commissioning functions, leading to improved services for patients and better value for money for the taxpayer. Strategic Health Authorities are responsible for:

- Developing plans for improving health services in their local area.
- Making sure local health services are of a high quality and are performing well.
- Increasing the capacity of local health services – so they can provide more services.
- Making sure national priorities – for example, programmes for improving cancer services – are integrated into local health service plans.

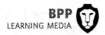

All Primary Care Trusts and NHS Hospital Trusts (other than Foundation Trusts) are accountable to Strategic Health Authorities.

Other bodies given 'Special Health Authority' status include:

- National Patient Safety Agency (NPSA – described earlier in this chapter)
- The National Institute for Health and Clinical Excellence (NICE – described earlier in this chapter)
- National Clinical Assessment Authority (referred to with regard to 'changes to staff ' in the NHS Plan in Chapter 13 and also with regard to adverse healthcare events earlier in this chapter)
- NHS Blood and Transplant (NHSBT). This is an integral part of the NHS. It manages the National Blood Service, bio-products and UK transplant
- NHS Information Authority. This is a special health authority that provides facts and figures to help the NHS and social services run effectively. It collects data from across the sector, analyses it, and then converts it into useful information. It was previously known as the National Case Mix Office. The recent priorities have been:

    - Patterns of prescribing and compliance with NICE guidelines
    - Supporting the patient choice agenda
    - To integrate NHS and independent sector information (support and guidance will be extended to private sector providers)
    - Using financial data more effectively
    - Widening the use of Electronic Staff Record (ESR) data
    - Improving and developing better social care information
    - Supporting SHAs with their information needs to answer policy issues
    - Promoting clinicians' use of information

## Payment by results and some other particulars regarding finance

The PCTs receive 75 per cent of the NHS budget. (The remainder of the monies are distributed to bodies and institutions, including arms-length bodies). For services which cannot be provided directly by the PCT, 'service level agreements' (SLAs) are arranged with providers. These arrangements deal with quantity and quality of provision, and are legally binding.

Historically, hospitals were paid according to 'block contracts' – a fixed sum of money for a broadly specified service – or 'cost and volume' contracts which attempted to specify in more detail the activity and payment. But there was no incentive for providers to increase throughput, since they received no additional funding.

Subsequently, the Government, through the NHS Plan, signalled its intention to link the allocation of funds to hospitals to the activity they undertook. It stated that in order to get the best from extra resources there would need to be some differentiation between incentives for routine surgery and those for emergency admissions. Hospitals would be paid for the elective activity they undertook. This in theory offered the right incentives to reward good performance, to support sustainable reductions in waiting times for patients and to make the best use of available capacity. The aim of Payment by Results (PbR) was to provide a transparent, rules-based system for paying trusts. It would reward efficiency, support patient choice and diversity and encourage activity for sustainable waiting time reductions. Payment would be linked to activity and adjusted for casemix. Importantly, this system would ensure a fair and consistent basis for hospital funding rather than being reliant principally on historic budgets and the negotiating skills of individual managers. Competition between providers would also be encouraged by this system.

The Department of Health consulted on its plans for introducing PbR in *NHS Financial Reforms: Introducing Payment by Results* on 15 October 2002 and published its response on 10 February 2003.

Presently, virtually all prices of services have moved from agreed prices and average costs ('national tariff') to PbR. Some notable exceptions at time of writing include critical care, although this

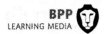

also has plans for shifting to PBR. The cost of healthcare varies across the country, just as salaries, land and house prices vary. The Department of Health therefore calculate the 'market forces factor' to reflect this variance and apply it to both PCT allocations and the national tariff.

## Healthcare Resource Groups (HRGs)

The Casemix Service develops and supports Healthcare Resource Groups, which are standard groupings of clinically similar treatments which use common levels of healthcare resource. The prime purpose of HRGs is to assist the Department of Health to implement the policy of Payment by Results. They also offer organisations the ability to understand their activity in terms of the types of patients they care for and the treatments they undertake. The activities which may be referred to include:

- Clinical governance/quality
- Performance monitoring
- Caseload management/review
- Programme-based resource analysis and allocation
- Costing and commissioning (this is accepted as the main priority)
- Enable the comparison of activity within and between different organisations and provide an opportunity to benchmark treatments and services to support trend analysis over time

HRGs are used as a means of determining fair and equitable reimbursement for care services rendered. These consistent 'units of currency' support standardised healthcare commissioning across the service. The current version of HRGs (v3.5) has been in use since October 2003.

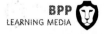

## Relevant questions – PbR

1. How relevant is PbR to your specialty?
2. Do you agree with PbR?
3. What are HRGs? What aspects of care in your specialty do you think HRGs will focus on?
4. Can you describe any problems that need resolving with regard to HRG/PbR and your specialty?
5. How could you help this Trust engage your Consultant colleagues and other doctors in producing high quality and timely discharge summaries in your specialty?

Satisfactory correlation between identification of the complexity of the outpatient/inpatient, the acute and chronic diagnoses in the inpatient, the interventions and the outcome (morbidity/mortality and discharge date) relies on satisfactory coding. Recognition of (and payment for) the activities of the Trust in turn relies on the timely delivery of the coded documentation (usually a discharge summary). In virtually all specialties, the outcome prediction, the clinical performance rating and tariff will be dependent on the entry of any complex co-morbidities for a given intervention (eg surgery or treatment of pneumonia). Omission of complexities in the acute and chronic diagnoses, and those of interventions and treatments, therefore may lead to an optimistic outcome prediction, diminished performance rating and diminished tariff. Trusts should therefore deploy systems which ensure satisfactory coded descriptions of patients, and timely discharge summaries. This will always involve doctors and coders working in partnership with other staff.

An age old problem which has not been satisfactorily resolved in all Trusts is 'how does the Trust engage Consultants and other doctors in producing high quality and timely discharge summaries?' The answer lies in the acceptance of the discharge summary (and its associated mandatory items ie diagnoses, interventions and HRG/ PbR correlations) as a non- negotiable product, and to make its production mandatory within a given time frame.

Although HRGs should not be seen as the omnipotent bible for quality references in clinical work, you can regularly refer to relevant HRG material while striving for clinical excellence in your specialty.

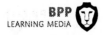

### Key points

- Be aware of the following bodies and philosophies: Risk; NHS Direct; National Service Frameworks; Patient Advocacy and Liaison Service (PALS); electronic data; NICE; Foundation Trusts; Primary Care Trusts; Strategic Health Authorities; 'Special Health Authorities'; PbR and HRG
- Remember: intricate facts are not important, though facts relevant to your specialty are!

# Section 4

## Important concepts and relevant bodies

Basic (not exhaustive) knowledge, and relevance to your specialty is important!

# Chapter 17

## Revalidation, appraisal, job planning and performance management

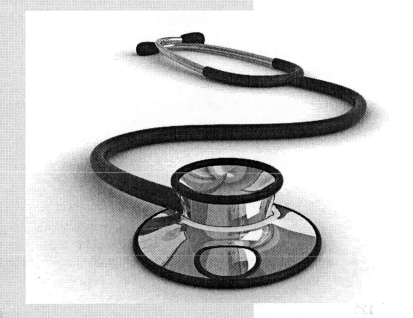

# Revalidation, appraisal, job planning and performance management

It should be remembered that the concepts of revalidation, appraisal and performance are often blurred and confused. Revalidation is a process which protects *the patient*. Appraisal protects the quality of training or career development of *the doctor*. Performance assessment *ensures service provision for the Trust*, although it simultaneously provides a vehicle for career development and therefore appraisal. The complex interfaces dictate that practice development cannot be assessed without any reference to performance or outcomes and performance management (including job planning) cannot occur without an understanding of practice development needs. *The concepts of revalidation, appraisal and performance are inherently separate yet interdependent.*

## *Revalidation bodies*

### A.    The General Medical Council (GMC)

The GMC was formed in 1858, and is the regulator of the medical profession in the United Kingdom. Its main purpose is to protect, promote and maintain the health and safety of the community by ensuring proper standards in the practice of medicine. It provides the licence for doctors to enable them to practise, and has the power to revoke this licence, or place restrictions on a doctor's fitness to practise. A practitioner not registered with the GMC is forbidden to present themselves as a registered medical practitioner in the UK. The GMC also contributes to regulation in medical schools in the UK, and liaises with other nations' medical and university regulatory bodies and their medical schools overseas. This leads to some qualifications being mutually recognised. The Council is funded by annual fees required from those wishing to remain registered and fees for examinations.

A registered medical professional may be referred to the GMC if there are doubts about his or her fitness to practise. These are divided into concerns about health and other concerns about ability or behaviour. Hearings may result in reprimands, restrictions on practice temporary suspension or erasure from the register. The processes adopted by the GMC need to have substantial agreement in principle from government and from many medical bodies (eg the BMA, the Royal Colleges). Over the years, the development of public confidence has been a priority.

The GMC also administers the Professional and Linguistic Assessment Board test (PLAB), which has to be taken by non-European Union overseas doctors before they may practice medicine in the UK.

The main guidance that the GMC provides for doctors is called *Good Medical Practice*. This summarises the standards and behaviours that are expected of them, and the document is at present being modernised, and mapped to the appraisal and revalidation process.

Subsequently, the government White Paper Trust, *Assurance and Safety – The Regulation of Health Professionals in the 21st Century* (published in February 2007) set out a series of proposals for further reform of medical regulation. The reforms proposed were welcomed by the GMC, who believe that they will lead to an improved and robust system of regulation.

At the time of writing it is imminent that the Postgraduate Medical Education and Training Board (PMETB) will merge with the GMC in the very near future. The decision followed a recommendation made by Professor Sir John Tooke in *Aspiring to Excellence: Final report of the Independent Inquiry into Modernising Medical Careers*. The merger will bring under one roof the regulation of all stages of medical education; this in turn may deliver benefits for patients and the public, as well as for the medical profession.

## B.    The Postgraduate Medical Education and Training Board (PMETB)

The PMETB is an independent statutory body, responsible for overseeing and promoting the development of postgraduate medical education and training for all medical specialties, including general practice, across the UK. It assumed its statutory powers on 30 September 2005 taking over the

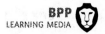

responsibilities of the Specialist Training Authority of the Medical Royal Colleges (STA) and the Joint Committee on Postgraduate Training for General Practice (JCPTGP). The PMETB's responsibilities include establishing, promoting, developing and maintaining standards and requirements for postgraduate medical education and training across the UK.

The PMETB is primarily responsible for:

- Establishing national standards and requirements for postgraduate medical education and training.
- Making sure these standards and requirements are met by monitoring, developing and promoting postgraduate medical education.
- Awarding Certificates of Completion of Training (CCT) and determine eligibility of doctors for inclusion on the Specialist and GP Registers.

The PMETB was funded by grants from the Departments of Health in England, Northern Ireland, Scotland and Wales. These declined in value until 2009/10 when the PMETB became self-funding. Income is now generated through various initiatives which include increased fees for CCT and applications under Articles 11 and 14.

Unlike the Specialist Training Authority (STA), PMETB is independent of the Royal Colleges. The STA is a body of the Royal Colleges whereas the PMETB is a statutory competent authority established by Parliament. However, the PMETB works closely with the Royal Medical Colleges by way of liaisons with their commissioning services.

Therefore it is clear that PMETB has dual roles in both revalidation and appraisal.

## Modernisation of revalidation

The paper 'Revalidation: a Statement of Intent' was agreed by the GMC, the Chief Medical Officers for England, Northern Ireland and Wales, the Deputy Chief Medical Officer for Scotland and

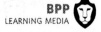

the Medical Director of the NHS in England. The plan at time of writing is to test and pilot, and have the process ready by late 2012. The aim is to develop a robust and standardised appraisal process (described below), which would require sign-off by the Trust's 'responsible officer'. Every fifth year, the sign-off would lead to revalidation. During the years in between, the doctor would annually re-validate using the process similar to that being used at present: that is, the doctor would not need to have any significant negative reports from the responsible officer, not be involved in any ongoing fitness-to-practise GMC issues, and by paying the annual fee. There will be following outcomes in revalidation:

- No registration
- Simple registration
- Relicensing (legal privileges) for all doctors
- Recertification (relicensing for those on Specialist and GP Register) – this will probably be deleted and merged with relicensing

## *Appraisal processes*

### A.   Record of In-Training Assessment (RITA)

The purpose of a RITA is to record the annual review of trainee progress through training programmes towards CCST/CCT. They are becoming superseded by the ARCP (see below). The main functions of the RITA are to:

- Ensure the trainees have had appraisals and feedback from their educational supervisors
- Review the accuracy of the proposed CCST date
- Check the completeness of the logbook/training record
- Plan the next year of training
- Provide career advice
- Review the quality of training posts
- Review the duty rota

*The panel members are:*
- Postgraduate Dean (or representative)
- Training Programme Director/STC Chair
- Regional advisor or specialty advisor

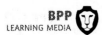

- External assessor
- University trainer (for clinical academic trainees)

---

*Relevant questions – appraisals*

1. Has the previous year been useful from a training perspective?
2. What were the good/bad points?
3. Were there adequate opportunities to increase skills?
4. Was there adequate supervision?
5. Was there sufficient time for private study?
6. Were necessary facilities readily available?

---

*The following points may be addressed by the panel*

1. What competencies are still required?
2. How and where is this to be arranged?
3. How will the trainee's needs be accommodated in conjunction with those of other trainees?
4. Are there any particular problems that need to be addressed?

---

There is usually scope for confidential feedback, and there is a vehicle for appeal if the trainee is not satisfied with the process.

At the time of writing, there are very few trainees still involved in RITAs, which have been replaced by an updated process, termed the Annual Review of Competence Progression (ARCP).

## B. Annual Review of Competence Progression (ARCP)

This has replaced the RITA process, and is also therefore an important process in gaining accreditation. It was conceived as an updated formalised assessment of a trainee's progress towards the achievement of a CCT (Certificate of Completion of Training). It has to be a transparent process, capable of standing up to public scrutiny. To achieve this, senior colleagues within each specialty have defined criteria, based upon the relevant curricula. At the time of the ARCP meeting, the progress of the trainee is set against this set of pre-defined criteria. In turn, this will be recorded regionally

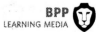

and at the Royal College to which the trainee will ultimately be recommended as a doctor who has reached a standard compatible with independent practice.

## C. Appraisal systems for Consultants

The term 'appraisal' should not be confused with 'revalidation' or 'performance management'. While the general public is protected by revalidation (see 'GMC' above), and the employer receives value by way of performance management, appraisals should be seen as vehicles to protect the practice development for the Consultant (and training for the trainee – see 'RITA'). This is an opportunity for the Consultant to meet with a peer to set objectives and improve the quality of career development. Nevertheless, it should be recognised that the revalidation modernisation process has created stronger links between the concepts of performance, safety and appraisal. Therefore, performance issues (including job planning) are given more attention in the modern appraisal.

Appraisals may occur at any frequency, and they may be formal or informal. The minimum requirement is for Consultants to be appraised annually and formally. The appraiser therefore needs to be an individual with knowledge of the concept of practice development, and a basic understanding of the requirements for development. It need not therefore be a Clinical Director, Lead Clinician or indeed a colleague from within the same specialty as the appraisee. Indeed, it may be an option for the appraiser not to be linked to Trust management, to avoid confusing the issue of practice development with those of service provision for the Trust. As mentioned in the previous paragraph however, the appraiser, irrespective of his or her identity, will need to be in possession of performance issues (fed from the clinical director) which impact on revalidation.

| | Appraisee | Appraiser |
|---|---|---|
| **Pre-appraisal** | 1. Collation of supporting information for portfolio<br>2. Self-assessment of portfolio<br>3. Presentation of portfolio ideally 2 weeks before appraisal meeting | Review of portfolio supporting information |
| **During appraisal** | 1. Reflection (break)<br>2. Refinement (strengths and development needs) | Refinement (strengths and development needs) |
| **End of appraisal** | Production of PDP | Completion of the four statements for revalidation |

**Table 17.1 Proposed appraisal preparation and practice**

| Domain | Attribute | |
|---|---|---|
| **Domain 1**<br>Knowledge, skills and performance | 1.<br>2.<br><br>3. | Maintain professional competence<br>Apply knowledge and experience to practice<br>Keep clear, accurate and legible records |
| **Domain 2** Safety and quality | 4.<br><br>5.<br>6. | Put systems into place to protect patients and improve care<br>Respond to risk to safety<br>Protect patients and colleagues from any risk posed by your health |
| **Domain 3**<br>Communication, partnership and teamwork | 7.<br>8.<br><br>9. | Communicate effectively<br>Work constructively with colleagues and delegate effectively<br>Establish and maintain partnerships with patients |
| **Domain 4**<br>Maintaining trust | 10.<br>11.<br><br>12. | Show respect for patients<br>Treat patients and colleagues fairly without discrimination<br>Act with honesty and integrity |

**Table 17.2 Proposed appraisal framework: domains and attributes**

BPP
LEARNING MEDIA

| | Supporting information | Minimum required |
|---|---|---|
| 1 | Significant event review/case review | 10 (2 per year) |
| 2 | Formal review of complaints | All |
| 3 | Audit/data collection | 5 (1 per year) |
| 4 | Patient feedback survey and review | 1 (year 3 or before) |
| 5 | Colleague feedback survey and review | 1 (year 3 or before) |
| 6/7 | New PDP and review of previous year PDP | 5 (1 per year) |
| 8 | CPD evidence | 5 (1 per year) |
| 9 | Probity self-declaration and review | 5 (1 per year) |
| 10 | Health self-declaration and review | 5 (1 per year) |
| 11 | Other information defined by organisation | All |
| 12 | Review of all items in context of GMP | 5 (1 per year) |

Table 17.3 Proposed appraisal supporting information

## Behavioural issues interfacing with validation, appraisal and service provision

Clearly, there may be instances where an issue (such as rudeness to patients) may simultaneously impact on practice development, validation and performance for the Trust. In these cases, the appraiser should make the relevant recommendations for improved practice, and subsequently inform the appraisee that separate forums may be required to deal with the issues of validation and Trust performance. After careful consideration, a decision would be made with regard to reporting to the GMC. The Trust would also take a view in relation to disciplinary processes. It should be noted that during disciplinary hearings in the Trust, the doctor in question will be entitled to legal and union representation. This is a very serious scenario for the doctor and the Trust, and should not be confused with lower level performance management discussions held between the doctor and his/her clinical director or other medical manager.

Appraisals are always linked to job planning; the latter should ordinarily pre-date appraisal, to allow the appraisal process to work within the constraints of the contractual framework.

## Job planning for Consultants

It is important to be aware of the issues with job planning, even before applying to be a Consultant, as it is the contractual vehicle with which you will be delivering your services. All your activities will be bound within your job plan, which in turn will be reviewed at least annually by your Clinical Director.

Planned activities (PAs) are time periods (eg 4 hours in a working week and 3 hours in a weekend) allocated for work. They are divided into Direct Clinical Activities and Supporting Programmed Activities. Direct Clinical Activities (DCC) are activities relating to direct patient contact eg ward rounds, clinics, operating, other clinical work. Supporting Programmed Activities (SPA) are activities which do not relate to direct patient contact eg clinical governance, research, teaching. There should be evidence for all of this, as the annual job plan review by the Clinical Director is now designed to question the value of all the SPA activities. If value is not seen, the Trust may seek to convert the SPAs to DCCs. The BMA suggests that each Consultant should have 2.5 SPAs for a 10 PA contract; this is contested by many employers, and many jobs are advertised as either 8:2 PA splits or even 9:1 PA splits. It is outside the remit of this book to politically comment on the validity of splits. It should be understood though that all SPA activities have to be justified, and are not there 'by right'. Whether Consultants are able to perform their SPAs off-site is up to the discretion of the Trust and Clinical Director – it should be remembered that if the Consultant is performing SPAs from home, he or she should be contactable and able to come in at short notice. The SPAs are distinctly different from 'non-contractual' days ie days where the Consultant is not asked to provide a service – on these days, it is quite ethical and legitimate for the Consultant to not be contactable if he or she so wishes.

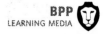

## *Relevant questions – appraisal and validation*

1. What is the difference between appraisal and validation?
2. With the proposed changes in revalidation, what issues do you foresee facing Trusts like ours?
3. What systems would you put in place to ensure or encourage Consultants to go through job planning and appraisal in a timely way?
4. If we were to appoint you, who would you expect to appraise you, and how often? What particular topics do you think you ought to be appraised on?
5. What should we expect from you, from your SPAs?
6. Do you think the present system for validation for doctors is satisfactory? Do you agree with the proposed changes?
7. Do you think that the current Consultant appraisal process is satisfactory? Is it just a 'tick box' process? How do you think we can improve the quality of appraisals for Consultants?

In response to the last 'tick box' question, it may be worthwhile considering the formalisation of CPDs, and clinical audit projects, with appraisal sign-off only occurring with strict evidence of the latter.

 **Key points**

You should be familiar with:

- The examples of appraisal and differences in the meaning between appraisal and revalidation
- The concepts of the GMC, PMETB, RITA and ARCP
- The proposed changes in revalidation for doctors
- The appraisal process for Consultants
- The methods for improvement of the Consultant appraisal process
- The job planning process

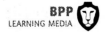

# Chapter 18

## Other important bodies and concepts

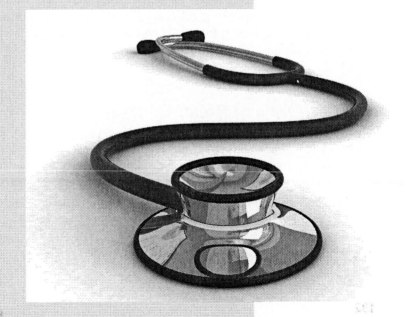

# Other important bodies and concepts

## *The British Medical Association (BMA)*

The BMA is the professional body to which the vast majority of British doctors belong, and owns the British Medical Journal, one of the world's more prestigious medical journals. It dates from approximately 1860, when it was established by the amalgamation of several regional medical associations. It allows doctors to be represented both by the geographical area in which they work, and by the various craft committees. The craft committees comprise (in alphabetical order):

- Central Consultants and Specialists Committee
- General Practice Committee
- Junior Doctors Committee
- Medical Academic Staff Committee
- Medical Ethics Committee
- Medical Students Committee
- Public Health Medicine and Community Health Committees
- Staff and Associate Specialists Committee

The BMA has sole negotiating rights for national Terms and Conditions of Service for doctors working in the National Health Service. It also supports public health initiatives (such as a ban on smoking in public places), responds on behalf of doctors to consultations by Government, and promoting the views and reputation of doctors in different arenas.

## *The Colleges and Royal Colleges*

The relevant (Royal) College will often issue information and opinions on current affairs, training and topics pertaining to your specialty. The interview panel will include a representative from the relevant Royal College (although this is not mandatory for Foundation Trust interviews). It is therefore important that you keep up-to-date with the latest matters and developments.

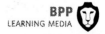

The College representative may deal with questions regarding:

- Modernising Medical Careers and the European Working Time Directive (see below)
- Training issues in general
- Controversies and political issues pertaining to your specialty

Although the Colleges play fundamental roles in overseeing medical education, and offer commentaries and visits pertaining to this, it should be recognised that the *Deaneries* hold the ultimate power for punitive measures000 if the Trust is found wanting. Nevertheless, if the relationship between the College and Deanery is close, the College may be able to exert indirect pressure on trusts.

## *Modernising Medical Careers (MMC)*

This was implemented by the government in August 2005 with the aim of providing a more consistent, structured, efficient and shorter training programme for junior doctors. The aim was that MMC would help facilitate the introduction of the European Working Time Directive (EWTD) into the working hours of junior doctors, by making the training more relevant and efficient. The shortening of the time taken to reach consultant level will in theory help address the shortage of consultants within the NHS, though some cynics feel that the quality of training is compromised. The old format of postgraduate training for junior doctors is gradually being replaced, and trainees of the new program will also undergo more regular and structured assessments of the skills they have learnt to ensure they are of the required standards. It is envisaged that these assessments will be conducted by a variety of professionals including consultants, senior nursing staff and communication experts.

The format comprises of:

- **Foundation Year 1**
  This is equivalent to the old style Pre-Registration House Officer year. The curriculum is based on the GMC's guidelines for *Good Medical Practice* and the primary aim of this year is to promote this practice

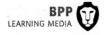

- **Foundation Year 2**
  This is equivalent to the old style first year of SHO training. In this year the curriculum addresses the doctor's competency in coping with a variety of emergency situations
- **Core Training**
  This has replaced the senior SHO/early SpR years. The length of this will differ depending on speciality but will normally be two years in duration and will provide an introduction to the chosen specialty
- **Higher Specialist Training**
  This has replaced the latter stages of the old style SpR training. The duration will differ depending on the speciality but normally be three to five years in duration and provide a more in depth training into the selected specialty

The introduction of MMC has caused great controversy and debate as to whether it will actually help to modernise the postgraduate training of doctors. The NHS Medical Training Application Service ('MTAS', the system to apply for MMC posts) has recently come against severe national and international criticism. The perceived over-complexities, the rapidity of introduction, the lack of protection of personal data were some issues. The system was terminated, and the Tooke inquiry was instituted in order to assess future planning. Contrary to some misconceptions, the inquiry has not recommended 'cancelling MMC' in order to revert to the training strategies of the past. The recommendations have broadly re-emphasised the role of 'core training' and 'higher training'.

| Advantages of MMC | Disadvantages of MMC |
|---|---|
| It provides a more structured training program to junior doctors especially in the earlier years of their post medical school training | Junior doctors are needing to make the decision regarding their chosen specialty after only two postgraduate years, and find it more difficult to switch specialties after core training, both as a result of procedural difficulties and also competition |
| There is now greater emphasis on training in the workplace, rather than purely theory | Therefore it is of concern that if doctors are unable to gain adequate experience in some specialties, they will be less inclined to embark on these careers, and these particular specialties will have a shortage of trainees |

| Advantages of MMC | Disadvantages of MMC |
|---|---|
| The training programmes will follow a set curriculum to ensure junior doctors receive a more predictable postgraduate education | Foreign doctors may have more difficulty in demonstrating competency in the new framework |
| It is producing Consultants about two years quicker on average than the old system | Some are of the opinion that the rapid escalation to Consultant level coupled with the restrictions in working hours posed by the EWTD will result in less experienced newly qualified Consultants |

## Relevant questions – MMC

1. What is your understanding of MMC?
2. Do you think MMC is a good thing?
3. What are the advantages/disadvantages of MMC?
4. How will MMC affect your specialty?
5. How would you ensure satisfactory training in your specialty?
6. Will future Consultants in your specialty be as equipped to cope as they are at present?
7. Has the Tooke inquiry changed the plans for MMC?

## Hospital at Night (HaN)

This was first proposed as a way of helping to comply with EWDT, and also maintain effective clinical care within the NHS. The project was first based around the concerns regarding the effects long working hours were having on junior doctors within the Deanery.

The aim of HaN is to have a multidisciplinary team which has the full range of skills to provide immediate care to patients at night and the idea is that the MDT can handle emergencies for a variety of specialties. The team may be co-ordinated by a senior nurse, such as a clinical site manager. This structure allows the reduction in numbers of junior doctors at night, without compromising the quality of care provided.

The HaN scheme was initially piloted in 11 hospital trusts in 2004.

The principles of HaN are:

- To give more responsibilities normally conducted by doctors to non-medical staff, especially nurses
- To reduce the amount of administration and duplication of tasks
- To increase the effectiveness of multidisciplinary teams which are assembled based on competency rather than grades

| | To patients | To doctors |
|---|---|---|
| Examples of advantages of HaN | Effective prioritisation of patients' needs through risk assessment | Improved teamworking during out-of-hours periods |
| | Increased co-ordination of care between medical, nursing and other staff | Reduced isolation of healthcare professionals and improved morale at night |
| | Allows the appropriate clinician to treat the patient in a timely way, without going through the irrelevant procedure of calling the 'patient's doctor first' | Reduced impact of long shifts on junior doctors |
| Examples of disadvantages of HaN: | Increased assessment of competencies are required. The relevance of recent specialty interventions are at times not appreciated by non-specialists (for example in a patient post-colorectal surgery, with an anastomotic leak leading to pneumonia, the pneumonia may be treated without regard or awareness of the role of the surgical issues). This may be overcome with satisfactory communication with the specialist teams out of hours and the following morning | |

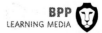

## *Relevant questions – HaN*

1.   We have an active HaN service in our Trust – do you know much about HaN? What are the advantages/disadvantages of HaN?
2.   Do you think HaN has achieved the goals it originally intended to?
3.   Is your experience of HaN positive or negative? Why?
4.   Has HaN improved the lot of patients in your specialty?

## *The European Working Time Directive (EWTD)*

This is a directive from the Council of the European Union to protect the health and safety of workers within the European Union. It lays down minimum requirements for working hours, rest periods, annual leave and working arrangements for night workers. The Directive was enacted in UK law as 'Working Time Regulations', which took effect in 1 October 1998.

The regulations place a legal requirement on employers and build on the progress already made through the New Deal. The regulations are also part of wider aims to improve the work/life balance for NHS employees.

The main features of the EWTD are:

• Doctors may work no more than 48 hours work per week (averaged over a reference period)
• Doctors must have 11 hours continuous rest in a given 24 hour period
• Doctors must have 24 hours continuous rest in seven days (or 48 hours in 14 days)
• Doctors must have a 30 minute break in work periods of over six hours
• Doctors must have four weeks annual leave
• Doctors' working nights must not average more than eight hours of work within 24 hours over the reference period

The EWTD initially applied to all workers with a few exceptions, including doctors in training. From August 2004 it was extended to apply to these exceptions. This has been phased in with a

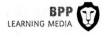

maximum hours requirement reduced from 58 hours (which was implemented in 2004) to 48 hours in 2009.

## SiMAP judgement

The SiMAP judgement refers to a case brought before the European Court of Justice on behalf of a group of Spanish doctors. The ruling declared that all time spent by residents on-call would count as working time.

## Jaeger ruling

The European Court of Justice Judgement on Jaeger followed the SiMAP line. The implications of the Jaeger judgement are that staff who are required as part of their duties to be resident in hospital or other place of work out of hours and who are provided with on-call facilities are considered to be 'working' during their period of duty. The whole of the resident on-call period counts as working time whether or not the member of staff is working.

Staff who are off-site, non-resident on-call or who are not required to be continuously present at the hospital or other place of work are not considered to be working unless called to do so.

## Diary cards

It is a common problem that junior doctors within one department or several departments do not achieve their requirements for EWTD with regard to length of shift or breaks during shifts. Human resources are obliged to issue diary cards when problems arise, and also when random diary cards are required. It is wise for all Trusts to invest time in interpreting diary cards in order to provide either a structured response to contest the findings, or the construction of plans to rectify problems. Ignoring diary cards may lead to severe actions from the Deaneries. Although diary cards help to substantiate rumours, they often cannot be formally acted upon if sufficient numbers are not filled in. Also, diary cards often do not answer the fundamental question as to whether the EWTD non-compliance is due to the fault of the department, or poor time-management of the junior doctor. Clearly, if the department is over-working their staff it should change, and if time-management is poor appropriate

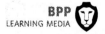

counselling and support should be provided. It is good practice for Consultants to reinforce with junior doctors that:

* Employers will never insist on prolongation of shifts beyond the required length
* All junior doctors should inform the team if their shift length is significantly prolonged or if they are not having their breaks, and the reasons why
* Junior doctors should feel empowered to stay beyond their shift for the sake of career progression, though this would be seen as voluntary

## *Relevant questions – EWTD*

1.  How has the EWTD affected the way in which junior doctors practice in your specialty?
2.  How has the EWTD affected the way in which Consultants practice in your specialty?
3.  What is your opinion on EWTD?
4.  Can you think of any innovations in your speciality which would allow us to implement EWTD better?
5.  (A scenario question may be asked with regard to junior doctors in the department working outside EWTD regulations, and identification of processes to identify and solve the problem.)

**Key points**

You should be familiar with the following concepts and bodies:

* BMA
* Royal Colleges
* MMC
* HaN
* EWTD
* Diary cards: their importance, uses and drawbacks

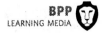

# Section 5

---

# Miscellaneous hot topics

# Chapter 19

## Medical education

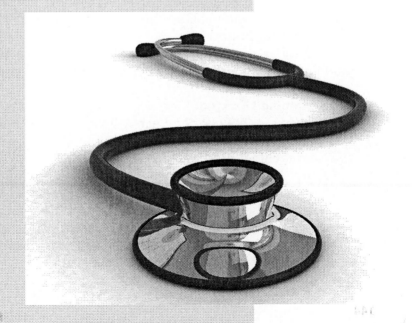

# Medical education

## *Training and education for junior doctors*

It seems fitting that medical education should be mentioned at this stage (after the chapter on medical bodies, MTAS and MMC). This theme will also be reinforced in a later chapter.

Not only is this topic vital for consultants and employers as a result of changing times with MMC and EWTD, it should also be recognised that sound medical education will lend credibility to your institution, and attract both deanery funding and quality trainees (and therefore in theory quality care). At present, Trusts are working very hard and are investing in personnel and systems to retain medical students and trainees.

The educational hierarchy is not used in the way it should in most institutions. The management structure (roles and responsibilities) are described here:

- **Consultant**
  All the clinical and education leadership skills inherent in the post
- **Clinical Supervisor**
  Clinical lead for education for that particular trainee; feeds issues to Programme Director and Faculty Lead
- **Educational Supervisor**
  Lead for issues such as career choices, bereavement and illness for that particular trainee; feeds issues to Programme Director and Faculty Lead
- **Programme Director**
  For example, Foundation Year 1, Foundation Year 2, Acute Care Common Stem (ACCS); feeds issues to Director of Postgraduate Education
- **Faculty Lead within a Trust**
  One Faculty Lead for each specialty group eg gastroenterology, diabetes/endocrinology, colo-rectal surgery. These specialty groups will vary in their makeup according to the size of the Trust; feeds issues to Director of Postgraduate Education
- **Director of Postgraduate Education (DME)**
  Medical Education Lead for the Trust

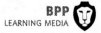

It is vital that clinical and educational supervision sessions with trainees are not missed, and that all issues are addressed in a timely way. This would reduce the chances of issues escalating to the Deanery. Deanery-approved e-learning competencies and courses exist to help clinical and educational supervisors.

It is common practice now for Faculty Leads to hold faculty meetings with all relevant educational and clinical supervisors in order to discuss issues, and for the DME to chair the Medical Education Committee attended by Faculty Leads.

Clearly, if issues are not addressed for the trainee by the individuals and committees described above, the trainee may need to correspond to the Deanery; in these cases the supervisors, Faculty Leads and DME need to be aware, and will need to have a sound working knowledge of the underlying problems, and how the Trust attempted to overcome these. Deanery feedback is very important, and negative feedback may lead to credibility and financial problems. The medical education team therefore will need to have real-time awareness of bullying and anti-social rotas amongst other things. Regular internal appraisals are required to avoid last-minute surprises.

Honouring shift lengths and protected time is paramount, as is the facilitation for practical procedures, which are allegedly becoming more and more difficult for trainees. You should always take refuge with simulation; the latter is now a requisite with Deaneries, and will augment clinical experience for practical procedures. Diary cards need to be understood. Persistent breaching of shift times may be a consequence of either inefficiency and poor time management, or on the contrary understaffing of the department. In order to combat staffing issues, you should attempt to achieve flexible manpower which reflects diurnal workload. Indeed, it may be worthwhile considering rotas with 'slight excess staffing' to allow the filling in for unforeseen absences and avoidance of ad hoc locums.

## *Relevant questions – medical education*

1.  What role do you think medical education plays in Trust strategy? (You should bring into play all the issues highlighted in this chapter)
2.  Are you aware of the medical education hierarchy? (You should demonstrate a strong knowledge of the roles and responsibilities of the individuals mentioned in this chapter)
3.  What do you think are the quality markers for clinical and educational supervisors?
4.  What are the risks of negative Deanery feedback?
5.  How should a Trust go about interpreting diary cards?
6.  How would you maximise medical education in your specialty? (You should be prepared to go beyond the 'usual' replies, eg ward-based teaching, simulation, and consider how your department could innovate to give junior doctors the opportunities to develop procedures and skills. For example, you could create departmental policies to prioritise procedures in favour of the less experienced doctors, or create novel ways of ensuring EWTD compliance and create internal/departmental appraisals to capture the problems trainees encounter)

### Key points

- Knowledge of the basic principles will maximise the functioning of your department, exercise the minds of the Trust and help differentiate average from good candidates
- You should know:
  - the educational hierarchy
  - the standards for clinical and educational supervisors
  - the risks of negative Deanery feedback
- Think about innovations for maximising medical education in your department

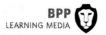

# Chapter 20

## Principles of leadership and management for doctors

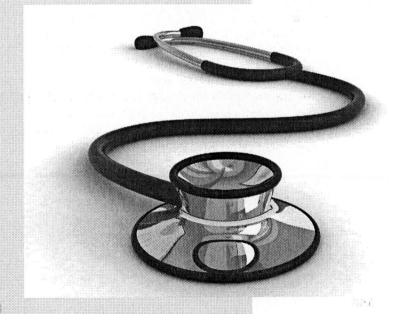

# Principles of leadership and management for doctors

Most scenario questions and psychometric stations will deal to a greater or lesser degree with leadership and management skills.

For doctors in the past, the possession of leadership skills were taken for granted. Authority was implicit in the job, and there were very few issues which the Consultant had to justify or fight for. Often, major decisions affecting patient care and finances would be dealt with whimsically, without recourse. Leadership courses were not perceived to be needed; to the contrary, arrogance was the main characteristic levied at Consultants.

These days, we live in times of numerous targets and standards which have been set by Government. These are designed to have the best interest of the patient and NHS at heart, and are clearly not negotiable at a local level. Here, a significant impact can only be made at regional or national forums. A key skill, therefore, is for the Consultant to identify issues which may be influenced at a Trust level, and to be able to use high quality leadership and management skills in order to achieve the best result for the patient and institution.

Key leadership attributes include:

- Motivational skills (happy followers are productive followers)
- Management of change and task completion (even if the followers are motivated, the Trust will fail if key changes are not made)
- Knowledge of political landscape (eg key governance/quality topics, mentioned in this book) to achieve goals
- Humility, courage, realism and passion are miscellaneous characteristics often possessed by respected leaders. On the contrary, leadership should never embrace victimisation

These attributes should be demonstrated in your portfolio.

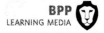

Although the distinction between 'leadership' and 'management' is often arbitrary, you should note the flavour of 'innovation', 'influence', 'inspiration' and 'vision' associated with the former, while 'facilitation' is strongly related to the latter. Clearly, many leaders are also managers and vice versa.

Most would agree that the non-clinical skills that incumbent Consultants and senior managers look for in a new colleague (and in an interviewee) involve management and leadership awareness. This is reflected in the nature of the questions. Topics already covered, and others yet to be discussed, include national politics, national bodies, financial structure, local Trust board structure, measures for standards, national and local finance, risk, complaints, ethics and legal issues. These are all 'management' topics.

## Management

Doctors of all levels of seniority, from Foundation Year to senior Consultant, have responsibility for running teams, departments, directorates or Trusts. They should all aspire to drawing upon available resources in order to play some role in setting and developing priorities, and to make other decisions to improve the provision of healthcare in a given situation. Therefore all doctors have an obligation to be aware of the principles of effective management and to work effectively in a multidisciplinary setting. Doctors are perfectly placed to provide management skills; they have the clinical knowledge around which most strategic decisions are made; often, one Consultant is able to formulate a management plan, whereas a handful of managers is required to achieve the same aim. Unfortunately, the converse may apply: doctors may make poor managers if they feel that 'they are too important to manage' or 'they are too busy performing clinical duties to manage'; the risk here is that unhappy doctors who do not engage in management duties are often left in sub-optimal situations without having the tools to improve situations.

## The GMC and management: definition and principles

The GMC definition of management in healthcare is:

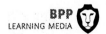

*Getting things done well through and with people, creating an environment in which people can perform as individuals and yet co-operate towards achieving group goals, and removing obstacles to such performance.*

The GMC also quotes seven principles of management for doctors:

1. Selflessness
2. Integrity
3. Objectivity
4. Accountability
5. Openness
6. Honesty
7. Leadership

## Relevant questions – leadership skills

1. Are you a leader?
2. What makes a good leader?
3. What leadership skills have you developed during your career?
4. What do you understand by the term 'leading by example'?
5. What is 'management'?
6. Do you think doctors make good managers? Why?
7. Can you recall a time when you had to demonstrate accomplished leadership qualities?
8. How would you approach an under-performing colleague?
9. What leadership skills would you use to improve standards in your specialty?

## Effective teamworking

Working as part of a team is vital for delivering effective treatment to patients. All doctors must demonstrate an appreciation of the characteristics of a good team and seek themselves to be good team players. The key points to working effectively within a medical team are:

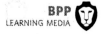

- Clear understanding of the overall goals of the team
- Clear understanding of your own individual responsibilities within the team
- Ability to clearly communicate with your team members
- Ability to listen to the views of the other team members

Many aspects of healthcare require doctors and other health- care professionals to work together. Effective teams are the means by which good, sustainable results are obtained. The medical profession has been increasingly keen to involve people from all clinical backgrounds in order to work effectively together in meeting shared goals for patients. As Trusts seek to become more flexible in the face of rapid change and more responsive to the needs of patients, they are experimenting with innovating and developing team-based approaches (eg Hospital at Night).

Many skills are needed for teamwork, including:

- Effective communication
- Listening
- Questioning
- Persuading
- Respecting
- Helping
- Sharing of effort and values.

## *Relevant questions – teamwork*

1. Give an example of how a complex clinical or managerial problem was solved through teamwork/deteriorated through lack of teamwork.
2. How many multidisciplinary teams have you worked within in the last few months?
3. Can you recall a time when you achieved a clinical or managerial goal through effective communication?
4. Tell us about a team you have helped to organise – what went well and what went badly?
5. Would you describe yourself as a leader or a follower?
6. What are the advantages and disadvantages of a doctor leading a multidisciplinary team?

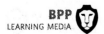

7. Should a medical team rely on one leader?
8. What is your opinion of giving nurses more responsibility in their role, in your specialty?

## The Medical Leadership Competency Framework (MLCF)

The Academy of Medical Royal Colleges, together with the NHS Institute for Innovation and Improvement published their own 'take' on clinical leadership in 2009 – a competency framework based on the concept of 'shared leadership'. There is an expectation and widespread agreement that the framework will be embedded in education and training curricula at all stages of medical education in the UK. Dentistry will no doubt follow suit.

The MLCF is not intended to be prescriptive, or indeed the final word on leadership, but it does provide us with a language with which to converse about leadership and a common sense of purpose in constructing training programmes or development opportunities. All clinical leadership development activity in the London Deanery will be mapped onto this framework.

Some Trusts use the MLCF framework for scenario questions and psychometric stations.

The main domains and attributes are as follows, and the challenge for each individual, whether they are Foundation doctors, core or specialist trainees, consultants or clinical/medical directors, is to make these domains and attributes applicable to them. Examples of actions for senior trainees and locum Consultants are in italics.

### 1. Demonstrating personal qualities

    a. Developing self-awareness: *innovate with multi-source feedback for a wide range of attributes*

    b. Managing yourself: *implementation in response to any feedback*

    c. Continuing professional development: *innovate in identifying forums for CPD (do not simply use 'courses'. Remember you can also undertake in-house CPD at your Trust)*

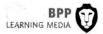

    d.    Acting with integrity: *deal with your own mistakes in a correct and professional manner and deal with under-performing colleagues*

## 2.    Working with others

    a.    Developing networks: *utilise experts in or outside your Trust to help solve a problem*

    b.    Building and maintaining relationships: *identify a network (or working group), and describe ways to keep relationships ongoing eg regular meetings*

    c.    Encouraging contribution: *innovate to maximise contribution (eg creating forums for good ideas) within a network or working group*

    d.    Working within teams: *display the teamworking skills described in this chapter*

## 3.    Managing services

    a.    Planning: *identify a new or adapted service and create a planning strategy, including a paper (including a business case if needed), network/group, obstacles, implementation*

    b.    Managing resources: *identify ways to define the nature, excess or lack of resources for any service and ways to implement any changes*

    c.    Managing people: *leadership attributes described above*

    d.    Managing performance and tackling difficult issues: *demonstrate awareness of political landscape issues (ie the framework of the problem eg appraisal, revalidation, performance/disciplinary) and implement the solution*

## 4.    Improving services

    a.    Ensuring patient safety: *for planning (see 3a above), itemise patient safety risks and make implementation plans to combat these*

    b.    Critically evaluating: *for planning (see 3a above), devise quality assurance (guaranteed benefits from the implementation) and ways of identifying problems or complications during implementation*

    c.    Encouraging improvement and innovation: *very similar to 2c; innovate to maximise contribution (eg creating forums*

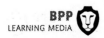

*for good ideas) within a network or working group – consider ways of creating similar forums for the whole Trust, not just your network/working group*

d.  Facilitating transformation: *try to get involved in practical ways to facilitate implementation of plans, particularly the hurdles/obstacles*

## 5.  Setting direction (strategy)

a.  Identifying the contexts for change: *for planning (see 3a above),publicise the reasons for making a change (including the risks of changing/not changing)*

b.  Applying knowledge and evidence to support such change: *for planning (see 3a above),use evidence to support your reasons for change*

c.  Making decisions: *demonstrate appropriate risk-taking in making a plan (3a), tackling difficult issues (3d) and overcoming hurdles (4d)*

d.  Evaluating impact of implemented ideas: *for example, for evaluating the impact of managing yourself (1b) or the impact on managing services (3) or the impact on improving services (4) – compare multi-source feedback before and after implementation*

### Key points

- You should be aware of:
- The relevance of history of leadership for doctors
- The fact that vital leadership skills for Consultants equate to main topics for interview questions
- The main principles of management
- The main principles of leadership
- What differentiates and unifies leadership and management
- The importance of teamworking and effective communication
- The Medical Leadership Competency Framework (NHS Leadership Framework)

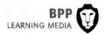

# Chapter 21

## The Trust management structure

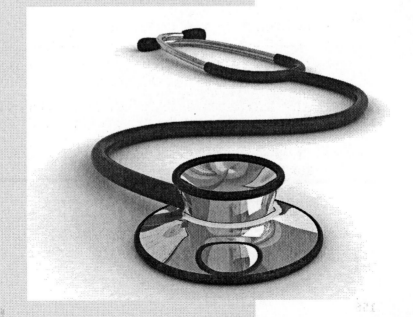

# The Trust management structure

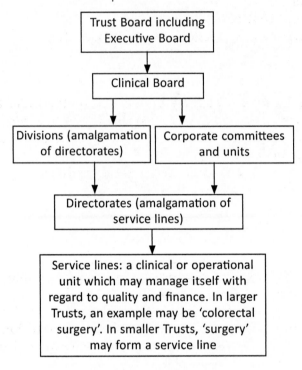

**Figure 21.1 The Trust management structure**

## *The Trust Board*

The Trust Board is the ultimate source of authority in the Trust and gives the overall sense of direction and purpose to the Trust's activities. It is headed by a non-executive Chairman, who is often part-time. There are in addition Governors and non-executive directors. The latter are drawn from the local community, and sometimes also from the Trust itself. The core group of individuals representing the Trust within Trust Board are the Executives (who also form the Executive Board).

Core functions of the Trust Board:

* Planning
* Standards and Performance

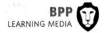

- Delegation: the right people in the right place to implement policies
- Finances
- Patient-centred
- Normally meets regularly (eg bi-monthly)

## The Executive Board

- The Executive Directors are headed by the Chief Executive Officer (CEO) and usually consist of the following:
- Chief Operating Officer (often doubles up as deputy CEO)
- Medical Director
- Director of Workforce and Communications
- Director of Finance
- Director of Information
- Chief Nurse
- Director for Estates
- Director of Strategy and Planning
- The Deputy Chief Executive will either be permanent or the role may be used on an 'as needs' basis

The Executive Board will meet regularly (in addition to Trust Board meetings), to react to Trust Board issues and also to focus strategies for Clinical Board

## The Clinical Board

This consists of the Executive Board, together with Clinical (or divisional) directors and divisional or directorate operational managers.

## The Division and Directorate structure (the 'middle tiers')

If the Trust board and Executive Board can be thought of as the 'top tier' of the hospital, and the departments (or specialties) are the 'service line tiers', the amalgamation or grouping of service lines (on the basis of some relationship to each other) are often called directorates, and form the 'middle tier' structure of the Trust, and their structures continue to rapidly evolve. If the Trust is large enough, the directorates are themselves grouped into 'divisions', 'business units' or other similar terms. Traditionally all doctors

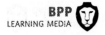

within the service lines, including Consultants, would be accountable to the medical manager in the middle tier (Clinical or Divisional Director), while 'everyone else' within the service lines would be accountable to the other figurehead, the Directorate or Divisional General Manager (also known as an 'operational manager'). These old values have by and large been superseded; it is recognised that the Clinical/Divisional Director should work in tandem with the Operational Manager, and be responsible together for all the staff in the Directorate/Division.

The Clinical/Divisional Directors (together with the Operational Managers) are operationally accountable to the Chief Operating Officer (though as with all doctors they are professionally accountable to the Medical Director).

## The day-to-day management of the Trust

This is often undertaken by Corporate Committees and units, which report to Clinical Board in the same way that Divisions and Directorates do:

- Strategic Investment Group
- Financial and Performance Review Group
- Operational Steering Group
- It is perceived that the Clinical Directors play a greater role in managing the Trust than previously

## Service Line Management (SLM) and Service Line Reporting (SLR)

A service line, as described in the diagram above on the Trust's board structures, is a clinical or operational unit which may manage itself with regard to quality and finance. In larger Trusts, an example may be 'colorectal surgery'. In smaller Trusts, 'surgery' may form a service line. For the benefit of the reader, it would be wise to simply see the service line as your department or specialty.

Service line reporting (SLR) is the act of reporting significant data from the service line to the tiers above (ie the directorates, divisions and Trust). The data will include those of finance and other quality items by which the Trust and departments are measured. For more

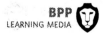

specific examples of reportable items, please read the chapter on quality and governance.

Service line management (SLM) is the methodology which allows the service line to become more autonomous in order to not only report upwards, but also use the reportable data to manage itself and forever improve. The theory is that local departments know what their staff and patients want, and therefore know how to use financial and quality information to maximise benefit for the patients and staff. Some academics see this system as the generation of institutions within institutions (or 'devolution' or 'local power'). It essentially allows departments to have less constraints from divisions and the Trust, and have the freedom to improve standards. Given this freedom, it is vital that Trusts give the Service Lines some framework within which to act ie basic lines which cannot be crossed and rules to obey, to avoid autonomy leading to failure of the service line and the Trust.

If SLM works well, the department with its local power should flourish, spend money wisely and be both responsible and accountable. The patients and staff within the department would feel secure that local people are making the right strategic decisions. One spin-off is that there would be a reduction in 'middle management' tiers.

## Relevant questions – management structure

1. Do you think that the 'Directorate' or 'Division' system works for your specialty?
2. Can you describe the differences in roles and responsibilities between the clinical lead and clinical director?
3. If appointed, how could you improve the profile of your specialty within the Trust Board?
4. Could you give us an example of issues that you would discuss with your Clinical Director/General Manager/Chief Operating Officer?
5. What do you know about SLR/SLM?

All management systems work well when the doctor and the manager know which aspects are 'operational' issues, and which are 'professional'. The former are discussed with the Clinical

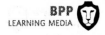

Director and General Manager (and if sufficiently important, with the Chief Operating Officer), while the latter need to be discussed with the Clinical Director (and the Medical Director if sufficiently important). As many issues have both operational and professional components, the Clinical Director is well placed to handle these, and to liaise with the General Manager and appropriate Executive.

Departments with good operational strategies (for example with regard to outpatient non-attendees, complaints and risk) work well and develop a high profile within the Trust. On occasions these strategies may need to be recognised by the Clinical Director, General Manager and Chief Operating Officer, and applied to other areas in the Trust, via the Trust Board.

**Key points**

You should:

- Know the board structures and their responsibilities
- Know particularly the roles and responsibilities of the directorate and division and their medical and operational managers
- Know the basic principles behind service line reporting (SLR) and service line management (SLM)

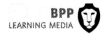

# Chapter 22
## Financial issues

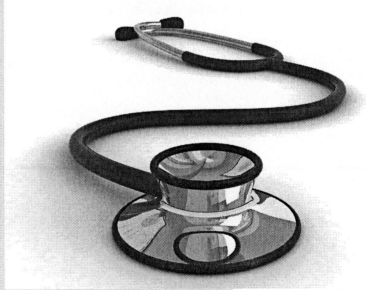

# Financial issues

## *General principles*

Although it is very rarely the case, all Trusts must aspire to all staff (not only budding Consultants) to be aware of the flow of money from the Department of Health to the specialty or service line. The amount allocated by commissioners should be understood, as should comparisons with previous years. Any payments made outside normal commissioning should be identified, as should the financial roles and responsibilities of the Executive Board and Director and Department of Finance. You should clarify in your own mind the role of the 'middle tier' ie the division and directorate with regard to financial gatekeeping and policing of financial handling by service lines. Finally, whether the Trust is performing service line management or not, the degree of financial autonomy of the service line should be established.

## *Executive duties: contracts for the Trust and understanding with the commissioner (Primary Care Trust or replacement)*

Long Term Service Agreements (LTSA) including a five-year plan are devised. This involves detailed discussions between the Chief Executive of the Trust, additional Trust delegates and PCT commissioners. Topics for discussions include:

- Standards
- Cost and volume of Trust activity (based on Healthcare Resource Group analyses/Payment by Results and block tariffs)
- The development of existing partnerships and integrated care pathways.

There should be transparent dialogue between the Trust Board, clinicians and users. Regular reports pertaining to the LTSA should be available from the Chief Executive. The latter should incorporate the strategy and annual plan, and prioritisation.

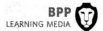

## *Divisional (middle tier) duties: gatekeeping and policing of service lines*

The Clinical/Divisional Director and Operational (General) Manager will try to ensure that financial safety checks are in place to protect the Trust from any risk from service line expenditure. The gatekeeping detail may be restrictions in the nature or amount of expenditure by the service line. For example middle tier authorisation may be required for any expenditure beyond a certain limit or any expenditure on personnel recruitment (irrespective of amount).

## *Service line (specialty) duties*

The service line should have a broad-angled lens when it comes to finance. It should look at income streams and expenditure, rather than 'a budget'. Maximising income streams by expanding services (or creating novel services) will become skill that more and more Consultants will need to have, as financial viability becomes a vital issue for all Trusts. Expenditure should be looked at in a systematic way. Broad categories include: pay (substantive and bank/agency), drugs, consumables and services (eg pathology, radiology). As mentioned in the chapter on management structures, the service line (department or specialty) is best placed to work out the best areas for diminished expenditure rather than the directorate or division.

### Key points

You should be aware of:

- The Trust and executive duties for finance
- The divisional duties for finance
- The service line (departmental) duties for finance

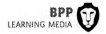

# Chapter 23

## Additional qualities required of a Consultant

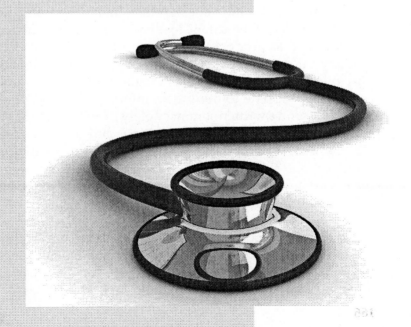

# Additional qualities required of a Consultant

## *Providing appraiser services*

As mentioned in a previous chapter, it is essential that the appraiser has a good working knowledge of what constitutes practice development of the doctor being appraised. An important question to ask is 'what can this trust do to improve your practice development?' It is not essential that the appraiser is a Clinical Director or a Lead Clinician. In fact it is perhaps an advantage that this is not the case, so that the issues of service provision and appraisal are not confused. However when appraising, it is important to recognise when an issue had an impact not only on appraisal, but also on revalidation and service provision. One example of such an issue is rudeness to patients. In these cases the appraiser should simply deal with the appraising issue, and organise further meetings to deal with validation and Trust management. It would be prudent for potential appraisers to attend appraiser courses.

## *Issues relating to discipline and revalidation of a doctor and colleague*

It is important to differentiate between issues of simple feedback (for example for minor substandard behaviour) and those for formal discipline. One-to-one feedback sessions should be seen by all concerned as productive. It is important not to label or imply that any informal feedback sessions dealing with difficulties are 'disciplinary', as the latter carries significant implications. It may even be appropriate to minute an informal chat and provide the individual with a written summary of this. In situations of a doctor's substandard practice, informal meetings and correspondence may become more common as all individuals and institutions have some responsibility to contribute to the practice development of the doctor and future protection of patients and other institutions when the doctor moves on.

When it is clear that the behaviour of a doctor will lead to a Trust disciplinary hearing, plans should be made. The meeting should be announced to the individual doctor, who then has a chance to be accompanied by legal and union representatives. The Trust

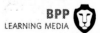

should make a decision as to who should attend this meeting; it would be essential to include those Consultants responsible for medical education (see previous chapter), other relevant medical personnel and healthcare professionals, operational managers and executive representation.

When there are repercussions with regard to a threat to revalidation, this fitness-to-practise issue should be dealt with by formal correspondence to the GMC. A copy of this correspondence needs to be sent to all individuals responsible for appraising the doctor. When a case is being assessed by the GMC, this needs to be declared at appraisals and interviews.

## Relevant questions – colleagues

1. A scenario relating to substandard practice in a colleague
2. What features in a colleague's behaviour would make you consider organising a disciplinary hearing, as opposed to an informal discussion?
3. What features in a colleague's behaviour would impact on fitness to practise?

## The Consultant Contract and job planning

Clearly, the practice development needs highlighted in appraisal meetings need to be reflected in the job plan; for this reason, appraisal and job planning need to go hand in hand. Both of these procedures need to occur at least annually. On the basis of appraisal if an activity is seen as essential, the job plan will need to accommodate by deleting other activities or expanding the job plan (and paying the Consultant more). On the contrary, if the requested additional activity is not seen as essential, the job plan is used to provide a framework and tool with which you can reject the extra activity.

From 31 October 2003, incumbent Consultants had the option of taking up the new contract or remaining on their current terms and conditions. All appointments to consultant posts first advertised after 31 October were offered only on the terms of the new contract. The aim of the change was to satisfactorily remunerate Consultants

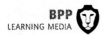

for the work they did in the NHS, while ensuring that the working time was carefully accounted for.

The new contract converted periods of duty (four hours during the working week and three hours during the weekend) into 'programmed activities' (PAs). An average of 40 hours per week, therefore, would equate to ten PAs.

The PAs would be divided into:

- Direct clinical care (DCC): this would include 'hands on' clinical care, including inpatient work, outpatient work and ward rounds. Many institutions allow DCCs for dictation of clinic letters
- Supported programmed activities (SPA): this would include general administration, clinical audit, education for trainees, self-education (translating into 'Continuing Professional Development' (CPD) points) and research

For on call work out of hours, the 'predictable' duties, such as weekend ward rounds and residential on call duties, are remunerated as PAs. 'Unpredictable' duties, such as being available for discussion and occasionally being physically present during on call, are remunerated as a (small) flat fee annexed to the salary.

Most new posts are advertised as '10 PA' posts. For purposes of cost and equity, there is a lot of pressure on Trusts to regulate the number of PAs paid to Consultants, and to confirm that the numbers are genuine. The usual recommendation is that 75 per cent of PAs are DCCs, while 25 per cent are SPAs. It should be emphasised that this breakdown is only an understanding, and often is not adhered to.

## Relevant questions – SPAs

1. Do you know much about the Consultant contract?
2. What is the relationship between job planning and appraisal?
3. How often would you expect to partake in Job Planning sessions, and with whom?

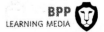

4.  What would we expect of you for your SPAs?/How can we guarantee value for money for your SPAs?
5.  Do you think it is acceptable that Consultants may engage in SPAs from home?

The point of these questions is the perception that many Consultants are paid significant sums of money for 'management', 'teaching' and 'reading journals', without there being any objective way of measuring output. This in turn may lead to resentment among managerial and other non-medical staff. The answer lies in creating a professional and accurate log of activities, such as timetabled teaching, meetings with managers and internal/external CPDs. Clinical audit projects (title, your role, status of project) should be formally logged. These details may then be discussed at the Job Planning session with your Clinical Director. It may be reasonable in the future that SPA's would be allocated purely on the productivity of these items, rather than there being an 'automatic' allocation which is perceived to belong to the Consultant 'by right'. Some Trusts are quite relaxed about the engagement of SPAs from home, on the understanding that productivity is guaranteed.

## Standards of business conduct

All doctors should act in their patients' interests, and this should supersede all other interests. They should be impartial, and there should never be an abuse of position.

Gifts should never be acceptable in order to induce action. When gifts are accepted, these should be logged with the General Manager. Money is never acceptable. Hospitality (for instance from the pharmaceutical industry) should be broadly similar to Trust quality. If this is not, the offer should be logged or declined. Where there is Commercial sponsorship for meetings or posts, there should be no inducement for the purchase of relevant products.

All doctors should declare any involvement with services which compete with the Trust, and also any outside employment/interest which conflicts with Trust duties.

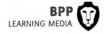

In the event that a doctor devises or invents a clinical product while in Trust employment, the intellectual property rights for the article(s) are transferred to the Trust. The inventor status remains with the doctor, and royalties for the article(s) may be negotiated by the Trust and the doctor.

Doctors' clothing has attracted a lot of debate. The public have, over the decades, become used to the pinstriped suit and the white coat. These days, however, where cleanliness and drug-resistant organisms are high on the agenda for the public and the Department of Health, it is not surprising that there are pressures exerted on the Trust by the Department of Health to review the clothing of doctors and Consultants. The initiative of 'bare below the elbows' is understood by many to be a sensible approach to clinical work to aid hand-washing; cynics point to the lack of evidence for patient benefit. This issue may become a very good example of a diktat which may only be negotiable at the level of Department of Health (that is, at Trust level it is not negotiable).

### Relevant questions – business conduct

1. Scenario question, pertaining to a gift/money from a relative.
2. Do you agree with the 'bare below the elbows' strategy?
3. How could you convince your colleagues to comply with the 'bare below the elbows' directive?

## How to develop a service or submit a 'business case'

It may be that an extension to a Departmental service is planned in your specialty. Indeed you may have been short listed as a result of possessing specific clinical attributes pertaining to the development. The panel will want to see that you are able to be a key player in these developments.

Even if there are no developments afoot, the panel will want to see that you will be able to submit a high quality bid for new facilities, taking into account the Trust's finances and predicament with regard to the PCT and other external pressures such as the Healthcare Commission.

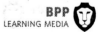

The quality of the background work (abstract and background) behind a business case should mimic that needed for a research paper. The basic principles are:

- Establish a case of need.
- Devise a business plan.
- Secure funding.
- Implement the plan effectively, with named individuals and roles.
- Review implementation for desired goals at agreed intervals.

Establishing a case of need can be identified by:

- Speaking to colleagues and gaining their opinion.
- Gaining feedback from patient focus groups.
- Analysing any recommendations drawn from previously conducted audits or authoritative external assessments.
- Comparing your new department's practice against others.
- Correlate with the Trust's pressures and anxieties eg patient satisfaction, inpatient/outpatient/surgical targets.

Once you have identified a case of need, a business plan for service delivery is then needed. A clearly presented business plan will be used by the decision makers in their considerations as to whether the proposal is credible, achievable and cost effective.

The business plan will:

- Explain why a service of this type is required.
- Justify why the service should be implemented.
- Clearly illustrate the cost versus benefits – eg reduce waiting times, save money, improve healthcare provision.
- If possible, factor in a risk assessment of implementing the service and not implementing the service.
- Provide a detailed step by step plan as to how the proposal will be implemented.
- Make recommendations as to who could fund the proposal. It is important that the plan is not seen as over-optimistic. There are three main funding options:

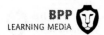

- Additional support funding provided by the local NHS commissioners (the local NHS Primary Care Trust).
- Monies from identified charities or donations.
- Monies released by closing or reducing a current service.

## Relevant questions – specialty expansion

1. How would you contribute to the planned expansion of your specialty?
2. What non-clinical skills do you have which would facilitate the development of your specialty?
3. What qualities does a successful business case have?
4. How would you contribute to establishing a new service, or an extension to an existing service, within the department you are hoping to join?

## Data handling

It is the duty of every doctor to use and handle patient data (electronic or otherwise) in a professional way. The Data Protection Act in 1984 suggested that all data should be:

- Relevant
- Accurate
- Updated
- Processed formally
- Not for disclosure
- Kept only as long as necessary
- Accessible to the patient who has eventual rights to access and amendment
- Secure

As mentioned in a previous chapter, each Trust should have named custodian(s) to ensure confidentiality. There should be strict terms of internet usage with relevance to context, browsing and software. On applying security, there should be appropriate facilities for data storage and passwords. Patient access should be facilitated by an application in writing to the Data Protection Co-ordinator of the Trust. It should be remembered that it also applies to information about health care professionals, research projects and corporate issues.

# Joint Guidance on Protecting Electronic Patient Information from the BMA and NHS Connecting for Health (CFH)

- Everyone in the NHS has a responsibility to understand the implications of dealing with electronic patient data
- Signpost key guidance so that each individual and organisation is aware of their responsibilities in protecting patient information.

1. **The NHS Code of Confidentiality**
   - Always log-out of any computer system or application when work on it is finished and do not leave a terminal unattended and logged in
   - Do not share logins with other people and do not reveal passwords to others
   - Change passwords at regular intervals and avoid using obvious passwords
   - Always clear the screen of a previous patient's information before seeing another
   - Use a password-protected screensaver to prevent casual viewing of patient information by others

2. **Organisational responsibilities**
   - Each organisation should have security, information, governance and records management policies in place, which should be endorsed by the Board or senior partners and updated at regular intervals
   - Organisations must complete the Information Governance Toolkit which measures progress against a series of standards
   - Each organisation is also required to complete an information governance statement of compliance, which ensures that organisations that use NHS CFH services meet certain standards
   - Organisations must ensure that staff are aware of good practice with regard to security
   - Staff members should receive regular training including:
     - What information they are using, how it should be used and how it should be protectively handled,

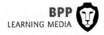

stored and transferred, including outputs from computer systems

- What procedures, standards and protocols exist for the sharing of information with relevant others and on a 'need to know' basis
- How to report a suspected or actual breach of information security within the organisation, or to an affected external information service provider or to a partner organisation

3. **NHS Connecting for Health's Responsibilities**
   - Smartcards
     Access to the NHS Care Records Service will eventually only be possible using a Smartcard and an alpha numeric pass code
   - Legitimate relationships
     Patient records should only be accessed by those with a legitimate relationship
   - Role-based access
     The elements of a record, which can be accessed, will be dependent on the role of the staff member and this is set up on registration
   - Audit trails and alerts
     Access to the NHS Care Records Service will be audited and alerts will be triggered to highlight possible inappropriate access

4. **NHS responsibilities**
   - The NHS Care Record Guarantee provides a commitment that the patient's records will be used in ways that respect
   - Their rights to secure, confidential and accurate record
   - There are 12 commitments, which include:
     - Records will be shared with healthcare teams on a 'need to know' basis
     - Identifiable healthcare information will not be shared with other government agencies unless permission has been granted, it is required by law, or approval has been granted for health or research purposes under section 251 of the NHS Act 2006

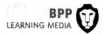

- Agreement will be obtained before sharing information with other external organisations such as social services or education
- Patients can limit how their information is shared

## Freedom of Information Act (2000)

This received Royal Assent on 30 November 2000. It gave a right of access to all types of recorded information held by public authorities and placed obligations on public authorities to disclose information, subject to a range of exemptions. In common with other public bodies, NHS Professionals were required to implement the Act fully from January 2005, when access rights came into force. This enabled anyone to make a request for information, although the request had to be in writing (letter, fax or email). The Act gave applicants two related rights: the right to be told whether the information exists, and the right to receive the information within 20 working days, where possible in the manner requested.

### Relevant questions – patient data

1. How would you ensure that patient data was adequately protected?
2. Can you identify any problems with data handling in your specialty?
3. How could you improve your service using electronic patient data?
4. There may be a scenario concerning transferring patient data using non-institution email services
5. Do you think that the Freedom of Information Act has benefited patients and healthcare professionals in your specialty?

## Dealing with the media

All issues relating to the involvement and presence of media within the Trust must be discussed with the Press and Communication Department in the Trust. This applies not only to VIP visits but also to the involvement of professional groups such as Royal colleges.

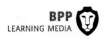

The trust must ensure that patient consent is achieved when appropriate. High profile patients must be afforded the same dignity and confidentiality given to all other patients.

**Key points**

You should be aware of:

- The principles of appraising
- The issues relating to discipline and validation of doctors and colleagues
- The Consultant Contract and the principles of job planning
- Standards of business: behaviour, gifts, attire
- Ways of developing a service and submitting a business case
- Patient data handling
- Ways of dealing with the media

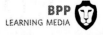

# Chapter 24

## Clinical governance and quality

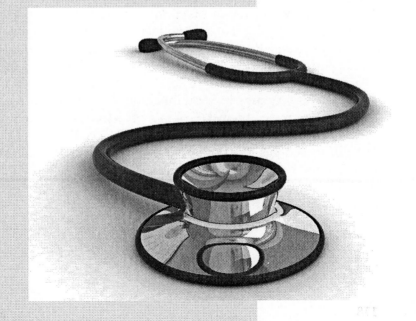

# Clinical governance and quality

Many of the topics mentioned in this chapter will have been dealt with in a slightly different aspect in other chapters in this book.

Although clinical governance in the NHS has probably existed in some form or another for decades, its history probably formally began in 1998 when the Department of Health published *A first class service: quality in the NHS*. This set out for the first time the Government's policy of raising quality for NHS patients and services. The policy involved setting standards through the National Institute for Clinical Excellence and the national service frameworks, and monitoring standards through the Commission for Health Improvement, patient forums and national patient satisfaction surveys. Central to this process would be delivering higher quality services through better self-regulation and through clinical governance. *A first class service: quality in the NHS* gave a complex definition of clinical governance:

> *A framework through which NHS organisations are accountable for continuously improving the quality of their services and safeguarding high standards of care, by creating an environment in which excellence in clinical care will flourish.*

More recently the focus of clinical governance has expanded significantly in the light of reports such as *Organisation with a memory* (1999), the Kennedy report on Bristol children's hospital (2001), the Toft report on intrathecal chemotherapy (2001) and *Building a safer NHS for patients* (2001). These, and the launch of the National Patient Safety Agency in September, have mapped out the quality agenda in terms of the NHS plan's objective of a patient-centred NHS. In addition, the National Health Service Reform and Health Care Professionals Bill spells out even more clearly that in future professional bodies will have to focus on improving their systems to involve more lay people and re-emphasise their role in protecting patients and the public.

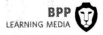

Key principles include:

- A framework for quality and standards in the right environment
- Accountable, safe, open questioning
- Relevance for everyone
- Important components:
  - Quality assurance, clinical effectiveness and openness
  - Risk management
  - Complaints
  - Clinical audit
  - Research and development
  - Education, training and continuing professional development

Although these components used to be thought of as 'pillars' of clinical governance, it should now be understood that every aspect of clinical work has an impact on, and is associated with, the concept of clinical governance. The risk associated with the identification and listing of specific components is that of misunderstanding the philosophy of clinical governance, and missing vital components which may not be on a 'list'.

Clinical governance is becoming such a popular topic that there may be many candidates who are now in a position to provide satisfactory stock answers in an interview. It is important to recognise, therefore, that interviewers are keen to identify candidates who are able to identify specific examples of ways in which any or all of the components in Clinical Governance may be used to improve standards for patients, the Trust and providers of healthcare.

In addition it should be noted that there are several meetings which encompass clinical governance; for instance forums dealing with complaints, risk, clinical audit and research are all technically 'clinical governance' meetings. This is often forgotten when asked 'How many clinical governance meetings have you attended recently?'

## *Quality agenda*

The term 'quality' could and should apply to every aspect of healthcare, and in this way it is exactly similar to the concept of clinical governance. Indeed, the terminology is slowly but surely changing to reflect this, and the 'clinical governance agenda' topics in healthcare is being replaced with 'quality agenda topics'. Every corporate body and institution, from the Department of Health, through the Strategic Health Authorities, to the Trust and its separate tiers (see the chapter on management structure) has a quality agenda. The clinical governance meetings for divisions, directorates and service lines are now in many institutions being renamed 'quality meetings'.

As mentioned in the chapter on management structure, it is vital that all the topics about to be discussed in this chapter which form the quality agenda (clinical governance agenda) of the Trust, divisions, directorates and service lines/departments (ie the tiers) are understood in the following way:

- Why is the topic important to the Department of Health, and how did the DoH go about creating strategies and implementation?
- How is this policed by the Strategic Health Authority (SHA) or anyone else?
- How do commissioners cater for this issue? Do they financially incentivise and punish?
- What is the opinion of the Trust governors?
- What is the overarching opinion of the Trust? Do they accept the implementation ideas of the DoH and SHA lock, stock and barrel, flexibly interpret and innovate, or flatly reject? Which committees representing the Trust police this topic?
- What is the role of the division and directorate? Is it to simply police, or is it also to innovate and interpret?
- How much can the service line (department or specialty) innovate and be flexible in its approach to handling the topic, in order to improve the quality of the service line?

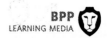

# Project leads, reports and meetings

## Project leads for each topic

It is recommended that each topic such as patient experience has a project lead at departmental level. This individual, which may be a doctor or nurse, should feel empowered to identify any problems and make necessary recommendations. It is still a rarity for Trusts to have project leads for quality/governance topics.

## Project reports for each topic

These should be constructed to summarise any recommendations by the project lead and focus on action points for the department for the topic.

## Quality (clinical governance) meetings

The positive comment is that many Trusts have numerous clinical governance or quality meetings in their various departments and directorates. The slight worry is that these meetings often have little or no impact. Discussion points may often not contain action points, and when action points exist, there is often little in the way of formal timelines for implementation. Most would agree that modern quality meetings should contain meaty discussion points based on the project reports (see above), and use time-based action points to improve the department.

# Topic 1: Patient experience and complaints

## Patient experience

Mandatory systems (patient experience trackers, PET) have been put in place in health institutions, to enable patients to input their experiences. The questions asked in patient experience trackers reflect the issues thought important by the government and also the local health institution. The results are regularly reported. High priority is given to the frequency of patient input (naturally together with the nature of input). The 'Doctor Foster' mechanism is at the time of writing the highest profile and most commonly reported tool for patient experience, though there is ongoing debate about how the DoH must be more flexible and adaptive to the needs of the Trust or GP practice in allowing a range of appropriate tools to report patient experience. In addition to the

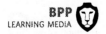

'Doctor Foster' tool, other systems also allow valuable feedback (eg 'message to Matron' on the ward, informal innovations such as feedback email and text facilities available to patients). Doctors have a huge role to play in managing patient experience; although traditionally nurses have been charged with developing these projects, it should be recognised that good professional habits from doctors will improve patient experience, while bad habits such as rudeness and arrogance will detract. Good experience will improve credibility of your department and Trust, and the commissioners will have an eye on this.

### Relevant questions – patient experience

1. How can doctors improve/lead on improving patient experience?
2. How can we measure or capture good habits and bad habits in order to improve?

## Patient complaints

Complaints handled efficiently should lead to quality improvement in the department. Reasons and causes for complaints include staff attitude, lack of information/ poor communication, poor care and lack of explanation of circumstances. The complaint itself is occasionally used to 'protect others' or manifest an expression of anger/grief. On occasions complainants may have raised expectations, be simply seeking compensation, or simply complain because it is now easy to do. Most would agree that the systems for complaints are better in these modern times; in previous years and decades vulnerable patients could or would not complain for fear of repercussions.

Complaints are either registered (written) or unregistered (verbal). Local Resolution (including meetings with complainants) held early should reduce the chance of registered and complex complaints. The process for registered complaints is as follows:

- Complaint received, registered and then forwarded to Complaint Lead (often the lead nurse for the directorate or division)
- Organisation of statements and investigation

- Draft letter by Complaint Lead
- Final letter signed by Chief Executive (or deputy) and sent to complainant
- 25 working days from start to finish

When the complaints lead seeks written statements from clinicians, the latter should be clear, in plain English, answer all issues and not be defensive. The clinician should apologise if there is a clear error and include actions to prevent reoccurrence. If the complainant is still dissatisfied, there may be repeated cycles of further explanation, further discussions and more attempts at local resolution. There may be further written correspondence. The final action a complainant may take , if unhappy with the process thus far is a request for an assessment by the Parliamentary and Health Service Ombudsman which is independent of the NHS and Government. The report and recommendations of the Ombudsman are seen as final. It should be remembered that the complainant may take legal recourse through their lawyer, even if the complaint is not upheld. The legal and complaints processes clearly have relationships, though no direct implications for each other.

*Relevant questions – patient complaints*

1. Are you aware of the complaints process?
2. How can doctors improve/lead on improving the department through complaints?
3. Have you been the centre of any complaints? How did you deal with it? Could you or the Trust have handled it better?
4. Scenario: a) a patient confides in you that she is upset with the conduct of a colleague (rudeness) – how would you deal with it? b) you receive a letter of complaint from a patient about your handling of a case in outpatients – how would you deal with it?

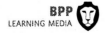

## Topic 2: Patient safety: morbidity & mortality, risk management and infection control

### Morbidity & Mortality ('M&M')

It is vital that all deaths, and all cases where illness could have been avoided, should be discussed in defined forums so that clinical practice may be improved. There have been allegations in the past that M&M meetings have simply been too relaxed, with no defined outcome. Appropriate cases should be entered in the risk register (see below), be logged as a serious untoward incident (SUI) or simply inform guidelines and protocols to improve practice.

> **Relevant question – M&M**
>
> If appointed, how could you ensure that the subject of M&M would lead to improvement in quality of your department?

### Risk management

This topic has been mentioned in the history chapter. The CQC ensures that the Trust and all directorates have registers of clinical and non-clinical risk (the 'risk register'). The items on the register are events which have occurred or are likely to occur, which may lead to risk. The project lead for risk for the department (which may be a nurse and/or a doctor) should report regularly to the department, and describe the risk profile and new items. They should also liaise regularly with the directorate/division risk lead to ensure that the reports are cascaded to the Trust. Protocols and guidelines should be regularly generated on the back of risk events, to improve the department. Risk should be consistently handled. Cross department/directorate/division learning is important within a trust. The NPSA (see history chapter) may be referred to for assistance, and on occasions certain reporting habits are overseen by the NPSA. The process of assessment for risk should be as follows:

- An electronic system is ideal – form goes to risk lead in department, nurse lead for department, clinical lead, directorate risk lead, and clinical director, together with a 'handler' (someone with expertise to lead on the risk event)

 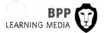

- Applicant(s) should be kept in the loop during assessment
- Regular interim reports issued to all involved
- The risk event is not closed off until the action points have been implemented

In the real world, the risk event is closed off quickly, as the Trust is under pressure to do so by the CQC. The solution is that even if the event is closed off by the Trust Risk Department, your own department can keep the topic 'open' locally until the action points are implemented.

Some other principles:

- Near misses should be included so that the department can learn from these
- The 5 × 5 matrix should be understood: a score of 1 to 5 for the chances of the risk event occurring, and a separate score of 1 to 5 for the severity of consequences of the risk event. The scores are multiplied to give an aggregate score between 1 and 25. It is standard practice for most Trusts to automatically enter a risk event in the risk register if the aggregate score is beyond a certain number. The 5 × 5 matrix should also be used after implementation of action points – the expectation is that the aggregate score is less post-implementation
- Some risk events may be entered on the risk register through sheer frequency, even if the consequences are not severe and the matrix aggregate is not high
- There should be considerable culture change for reporting. Risk is not a 'no blame' system but rather 'appropriate blame'; nevertheless fear should not take over, and reporting should be second nature to improve your department

*Relevant questions – risk*
1. If appointed, how could you ensure that the subject of risk would lead to improvement in quality of your specialty?
2. If appointed, how could you lead on risk reporting in your department?

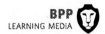

## Infection control

Doctors are not as intensely engaged with infection control issues as they should be. The project lead (usually a nurse) in your department should report on departmentally-acquired cases of MRSA, MRSA bacteraemias and *C. difficile* cases. MRSA bacteraemias and deaths related to infection control issues should lead to mandatory root cause analyses. Annual targets are set by the CQC for each Trust for MRSA and C. difficile. The Department of Health, intermittently with input from the NPA, have set a group of High Impact Interventions (HII), designed to improve infection control issues. These range from inspection of intravenous cannulae, central venous catheters, dressings and other items. It is usual for nurses to lead on these assessments, though it is clear that doctors' involvement is critical. Departments and Trusts may fail on infection control-related targets and standards as a direct consequence of doctors not being aware of the issues.

> *Relevant question – infection control*
>
> If appointed, how could you ensure that the subject of infection control would lead to improvement in quality of your specialty?

## *Topic 3: Research*

Most doctors, by the time they are senior trainees, have embarked on some form of research. The later may range from the simple submission of abstracts and posters in national and international seminars, submission of original paper to credible journals, to participation in high-ranking research projects and higher academic doctorates. As mentioned in the beginning of this book, high quality research will add credibility to the individual, the department and the Trust in the eyes of patients and commissioners. It is correct to say though, that other than the assessment of high quality research for academic posts, the simple issue of 'research' carries much less weighting for recruitment to NHS consultant posts than it used to. However it is also correct to say that an intellectual analysis of research activities, and their relationship to quality improvement and clinical effectiveness, is valued as highly as other 'management' traits.

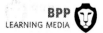

Research topics which will need to be prevalent amongst all Consultant staff, and which may be discussed in an interview, are:

- The mechanisms of turning 'evidence' into practice: peer review via local committee and consensus; creation of guideline/protocol; submission of accompanying business case if expenditure required; submission to relevant Trust committee for approval
- Examining the advantages and disadvantages of following national guidelines which the Trust is under pressure to follow, and articulating these issues. For example, the Consultant should be able to submit a paper on the reasons for not following NICE guidelines, where relevant

When embarking on any research, the individual, the Research and Development Department and the Trust will need to demonstrate research governance, even for the simplest case report. Research governance issues include patient consent for research, data confidentiality and patient consent for publication in journals. It will be a requisite in the near future that all researchers, including those simply submitting case reports, should have a certificate in research governance issues (as evidence of 'Good Medical Practice').

*Relevant questions – research*
1. How highly do you value research?
2. What aspects of research should we fund as a Trust?
3. Which of your research qualities would contribute to the improvement of your department?
4. If you were appointed how would you ensure the implementation of sound research governance by all your colleagues?
5. Scenario: you have recently read a paper (meta-analysis) in a credible journal that suggests that certain policies in your department need to change – how would you go about assessing whether this is the case?

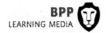

## *Topic 4: Finance*

Finance is another topic which most doctors have less than a working knowledge of. Allegations are often made that doctors 'will spend more money to ensure the benefit of one patient, while emptying the coffers of the Trust and thereby ensuring poor quality of care for most other patients' (personal communication). Even though it is the *highest* priority of any Trust to provide high quality care, it is also the duty of all doctors and particularly Consultants to ensure that standards are met within the constraints of budget. The ultimate penalty for financial mishandling is the downsizing of your department or even its removal.

The responsibilities of the tiers (Trust Department of Finance, division, directorate and service line/department) should be set. The Trust will set the framework and rules, the division/directorate will police the rules and oversee essential items such as overspend, and the department/service line should take responsibility for the bulk of budgeting. The departmental finance manager is usually the lead nurse, who liaises with the Lead Clinician. As hinted in this paragraph, directorates and divisions become involved when for example:

- There is a risk of, or there is actual overspend
- A change of strategy carries a risk of overspend
- There is proposed extraordinary expenditure by the department:
  - Capital (single spend, usually hardware or equipment) or
  - Revenue (recurrent spend, usually salary)
- Business cases are made

Average departments look at departmental finance and see a 'budget' (or simply expenditure limits). Excellent departments see income and expenditure streams, and have plans to maximise the former and minimise the latter. Income streams include:

- Maximising coding and HRG: it is essential that all diagnoses are correctly coded (usually in discharge summaries)
- Engaging in CQUINS (see below)

BPP
LEARNING MEDIA

- Expanding the capabilities of the department ie offer to provide a service to the commissioners which they are currently not getting from you

Expenditure streams, which need to be ethically minimised include:

- Pay
  - Substantive
  - Bank/locum/agency
- Consumables (perpetually-used hardware items)
- Other capital expenditure eg new equipment (a business case will have been made)
- Drugs (are the best drugs being used at the cheapest price?)
- Services (is the department using radiology and pathology efficiently?)

The finance project lead for the department should submit a report outlining any action plans for the items above.

> *Relevant questions – financial issues*
> 1. If appointed, what role would you be expected to play in financial issues in your department?
> 2. What major interventions could you make to maximise income?
> 3. How would you reduce expenditure?
> 4. Scenario: you have been told by your Lead Nurse that expenditure on a certain blood test has been top of your department's expenditure list for 2 years – how would you deal with this issue?

## Topic 5: Using the Commissioning for Quality and Innovation (CQUIN) payment framework

The allegation over the last decade has been that successive governments have been more focussed on targets than actual quality. In an effort to incentivise healthcare workers to achieve certain quality issues (and punish for not achieving these), the CQUIN framework was devised.

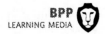

The CQUIN framework is a national framework for locally agreed quality improvement schemes. A portion of the contractual payment by commissioners will only be received by the Trust if CQUIN markers are achieved. Providers of ambulance, community, mental health and learning disability services using national contracts, like providers of acute services, now also need a full CQUIN scheme to earn CQUIN money. Commissioners must make 1.5% of contract value (at the time of writing this book) available for each provider's CQUIN scheme and CQUIN goals should reflect local priorities set out in the NHS Operating Framework.

Goals should be stretched and focused. Trusts will not achieve CQUIN money for achieving minimum expectations set out by other standards (eg CQC). Acute schemes must include the specified national goals (called 'National CQUINS or NCQUINS') that the NHS Operations Board confirm. In 2010/11, the NCQUINS were reducing the impact of Venous Thromboembolism (VTE) and improving responsiveness to personal needs of patients.

The CQUINS which are 'regional' ie locally arranged between the commissioners and Trusts are called 'Regional CQUINS' or RCQUINS. SHAs are responsible for assuring schemes and ensuring that commissioners and Trusts arrange schemes which demonstrate stretch and focus.

There will be a CQUIN relevant to your specialty, and you must be completely aware of what these are. It is reasonable for the department to have a CQUIN project lead, who reports on whether the department is delivering on CQUINS, and whether systems are required to do so. As in most topics, doctors may be occasionally responsible for losing significant income from lack of awareness of the importance of CQUINS. It is therefore important for Consultants to lead on implementation.

---

*Relevant questions – CQUINS*
1. Do you know what CQUINS are?
2. What are the CQUINS relevant to your specialty?
3. If appointed, what role would you be expected to play in maximising the income from CQUINS?

---

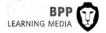

## Topic 6: Staff

It is always vital that a relevant member of staff in the department is responsible for all staff issues. This is particularly relevant for Consultants and includes traditional items such as appraisal, revalidation, performance, education and practice development. The Mid-Staffordshire inquiry further reinforced the need to nurture staff, and oversee any concerns.

Issues with health and sickness for an individual Consultant are normally dealt with in the annual appraisal (see previous chapter), though it is wise for the department to have one lead who is responsible for all Consultants. This is usually the Lead Clinician.

Scenarios in the department may include repetitive sickness in one Consultant; it is essential that this is dealt with in a professional and courteous manner. Action plans may include one-to-one sessions, recommendations to see Occupational Health, relevant specialists and the GP. 'Return to work' schedules should be devised by the Lead Clinician in conjunction with Occupational Health.

The Lead Clinician (together with the appraisal mechanism) would also deal with conduct issues (courtesy, professionalism, rudeness and unprofessionalism), and facilitate interviews including disciplinary hearings if required.

The Lead Clinician should also create a confidential forum for all Consultants to voice any concerns, and should make clear the formal 'whistle blowing' policy which should exist in the Trust, in keeping with national guidelines.

### Relevant questions – forums

1. How important is it to provide a forum for Consultants to voice their concerns, and why?
2. If we appointed you, who would deal with your health and sickness issues?
3. If we appointed you, who would deal with your conduct issues? What type of interviews or meetings dealing with conduct are you aware of?

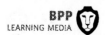

> 4. Scenario: you are asked by a fellow Consultant to prescribe him antidepressants; or a colleague is consistently turning up late for ward rounds and clinics; or a colleague has not dealt with CPDs for 5 years; colleague has voiced significant concerns for 3 months, and may be suggesting that patient care is compromised

## Topic 7: Clinical effectiveness including clinical audit

### Protocols, guidelines and clinical effectiveness

Clinicians and the public alike need reassurance that standards are being met; protocols and guidelines for departments and specialties should be designed to promote operational and clinical excellence. One definition of clinical effectiveness is the usage of tools (such as policies and guidelines) to maintain and improve clinical and operational excellence, the usage of clinical audit to evaluate these tools, and the usage of educational and other processes to learn and improve in response to clinical audit. Trusts will prioritise the adoption of some guidelines which will promote compliance with third party measurables (eg CQC).

NICE guideline compliance is increasingly measured. At present it is simply the Trust's response to the appropriateness of a NICE guideline which is fed back by the Trust back to NICE. In the future however, with the increasing prominence and authority of NICE, and the minds of solicitors and patients exercised, it is likely that NICE compliance will become mandatory. It is also likely that commissioners will look favourably at Trusts which are NICE compliant.

It is accepted by most that policies and guidelines help focus the mind of the clinician. Those who worry that their clinical freedom is compromised by policies will need reminding that systems will always be in place to allow variation in practice according to relevant circumstances, and that needless variation in practice compromises patient safety. Drivers for the production of policies, guidelines and protocols should be established in the Trust and adopted by your department. Ordinarily, the Trust would prioritise the conception of policies in the following order:

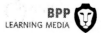

1.    National diktat such as NICE
2.    Local diktat derived from various Trust committees
3.    Risk event, Patient experience tracker/complaint, New research, Finance

There should be reinforcement of the concept of a tracker for policies, guidelines and clinical effectiveness in general. The following stages should be tracked:

• Conception of policy/guideline/protocol
• Driver for the policy/guideline/protocol (see above)
• Project lead
• Date of approval by Trust
• Date of implementation commencement
• Date of first clinical audit

## Clinical audit

Although most doctors including Consultants have a need to do clinical audit for their appraisals, anecdotally most see the need to do audit as a 'tick box exercise'. The opinion of this author as to the reason behind this is that the meaning of audit is often lost. You should remember that while performing clinical audit, you are invariably comparing performance against a standard (or policy/guideline/protocol). Your department therefore needs a policy/guideline/protocol! This fact is often lost on individuals. If doctors could see that the creation of policies, and then timely auditing, could improve their department, many would start at the beginning of the process and examine the policies and guidelines required by their department. Clinical audit is important, but clinical effectiveness is the key. The creation of policies followed by clinical audit would look far better in a CV than a standalone audit.

The drivers for clinical audit should have the same priorities as described for policies and guidelines, and the date and timing for audit should have been scheduled when the policy/guideline was ratified (see above). A proposed date for audit could be brought forward if for instance:

• You have a personal experience or view that things could be done better
• An adverse event occurs
• A complaint is made

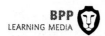

It is recommended that the Trust has one forum for presentations of clinical audit, so that these may be logged and action (implementation) points recorded.

Tried and variably-trusted techniques for implementation of findings from clinical audit include:

- Feedback
- Educational strategies
- Materials
- Conferences/seminars/workshops
- Outreach visits by opinion leaders to Trusts, Departments and Directorates
- Patient mediated. The strength and potential of this has not been widely implemented
- Self-efficacy: involvement of those who have a perception of 'lack of knowledge', together with practical support
- Inverse social facilitation: for those individuals thought not to care ('social loafers, free-riders'), make them accountable
- Reminders
- Organisational change
- Combination of any or all of the above

## Re-audit date
This should be set at the time of presentation.

*Relevant questions – audit*
1. Why do you think clinical audit is thought to be so important?
2. What is your definition of clinical effectiveness?
3. Do you think that policies and guidelines are beneficial or detrimental? Can there be too many policies and guidelines?
4. A collection of junior doctors in your department want to perform clinical audit – how would you prioritise/schedule projects?

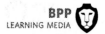

**Key points**

You should:

- Know the history and philosophy of clinical governance and quality
- Know the important components of quality improvement: patient experience and complaints; patient safety (M&M, risk, infection control); research and research governance; finance; CQUIN; staff; and clinical effectiveness, including clinical audit
- If asked about clinical governance/quality in an interview, try to think of specific examples where interventions may improve standards
- Be aware of the key individuals and Trust committees that deal with topics important to clinical governance (eg risk, complaints, clinical audit, research, training/education)
- Be prepared to volunteer to run regular clinical governance/ quality meetings in your department/specialty

# Chapter 25

## Continuing education and development

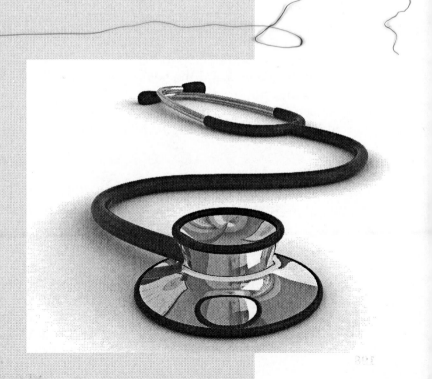

# Continuing education and development

It is no longer considered acceptable for doctors to ignore the need to continue their education and development, even after achieving Consultant status. After the years of training it is possible to feel, with genuine conviction, that you know 'enough' to do the job. However, hypotheses and intellectual viewpoints change, as does clinical evidence. The drive for clinical effectiveness is never-ending, and this may only be achieved with a good working knowledge of evidence-based medicine and an awareness of clinical controversies and issues. The Chief Medical Officer for England has emphasised the need for lifelong learning to meet patients' needs and deliver NHS priorities. Therefore the government has identified this as a key responsibility of NHS Trusts; there is an earmarked budget designed to support this process. The whole medical infrastructure relies on doctors helping to train and teach their peers and junior colleagues. It is vital therefore that doctors show passion and enthusiasm for teaching. It is also important that all medical educators take a broad view about the topics that should be included in medical education. In addition to the accepted academic content, it may be essential to include the following topics in order to improve medical outcome:

- Management
- Corporate and political topics
- Healthcare ethics and the law
- Communication skills
- Information technology skills
- Skills in teaching, research, interviewing, and committee work

## *Continuing Professional Development (CPD)*

This is the means by which doctors improve and broaden their knowledge and skills and develop the personal qualities required in their professional lives. In addition it is a vehicle for doctors to take responsibility for their own ongoing development, the evidence of which will form the basis of appraisal (and eventually also validation, where the public can be assured that the doctor's education correlates with fitness to practise). It is a systematic and coherent approach to education. The medical Royal Colleges set

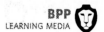

standards for yearly CPD achievements and award educational courses time-based credits. Many strategies may be used to acquire CPDs; these may include reflective practice, audit, portfolio development and multidisciplinary cooperation. The goal is the promotion of a culture in which doctors retain a curiosity about their subject that is a stimulant for lifelong learning.

Some characteristics of teaching include:

- Enthusiasm and passion
- Clear communication skills
- Sound knowledge base
- Ability to listen to and assess your students' learning progress
- Use of clear teaching materials
- Use of case studies to bring an applied approach to your teaching

## Problem-based learning (PBL)

This is an educational, academic concept of 'active learning' in tertiary education, especially within medicine. It was pioneered and used extensively at McMaster University, Hamilton, Ontario, Canada. Some defining characteristics of PBL are:

- Learning that is driven by challenging, open-ended problems
- Students working in small collaborative groups
- Teachers taking on the role as 'facilitators' of learning; students are encouraged to take responsibility for their group and to organise and direct the learning process with support from a tutor or instructor
- A PBL cycle concludes with reflections on learning, problem solving, and collaboration
- A structured system is used to help the learners keep track of their problem solving and learning
- Feedback and reflection on the learning process and group dynamics are essential

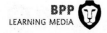

Advocates of PBL claim it can be used to enhance content knowledge and foster the development of communication, problem-solving and self-directed learning skills.

## Relevant questions – CPD

1. Why do you think continuing medical education is important?
2. What is CPD? / What are the benefits of CPD? / How should CPD be regulated?
3. How could you make education for your peers and junior staff more efficient?
4. Talk us through your teaching experience.
5. What makes you a good teacher?
6. How do you assess competence for a given procedure in a colleague?
7. What do you consider to be the most effective form of teaching?
8. What is problem-based learning? What are the advantages and disadvantages?

### Key points

You should be aware of;

- The importance of continuing education
- CPD
- Characteristics of good teaching
- PBL

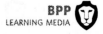

# Chapter 26

## Legal and ethical issues

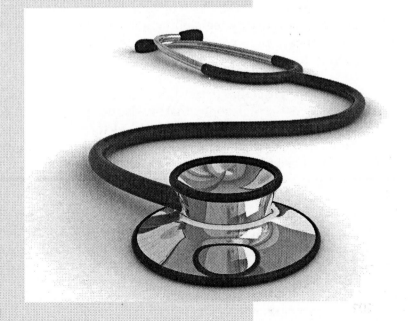

# Legal and ethical issues

Legal and ethical issues impact daily on our medical lives. Topics include:

- Assessing the capacity of a patient
- Seeking consent
- The non-commencement or withholding of medical treatment
- End-of-life care
- Adverse incidents and medical error; implications for legal action and the sharing of information with patients and relatives
- Complaints and the implications for legal action

## *Assessing the capacity of a patient and the Mental Capacity Act (MCA)*

The Mental Capacity Act 2005 has been fully in force since October 2007. This clarified the law with regard to dealing with the incapacitated patient, and codified the law with regard to best interests. It introduced the concept of substituted decision-making and placed advance refusals on a statutory footing. Lasting Powers of Attorney (LPA) were introduced as was the Independent Mental Capacity Advocate (IMCA). The aim was to introduce a code of practice to accompany legislation, and did not apply to treatment for mental disorders which would within the remit of the Mental Health Act.

The MCA suggests that there should be a presumption of capacity and reinforces the philosophy that unwise decisions should not imply that the patient is incapable. Any acts performed on incapacitated patients must be in their best interests, and there should be an assessment as to whether a less restrictive option may achieve the clinical purpose.

The patient lacks capacity if he or she is unable to make a decision for himself or herself because of impairment of, or disturbance in the functioning of, the mind or brain. This impairment may be permanent or temporary. The focus should be on the particular

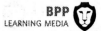

matter and the particular time when a decision has to be made. The principle should be of equal consideration – the decision should not be based on age, appearance or unjustified assumptions.

The patient may be seen to be unable to make a decision if on balance of probabilities he or she is unable to:

- Understand the information relevant to the decision (as presented appropriately and with assistance)
- Retain that information (long enough to make a choice or decide)
- Use or weigh that information as part of the process of making the decision
- Communicate his or her decision

The person making the determination must consider all relevant circumstances and take the following steps (except in the case for advance refusals):

- Consider whether the patient will regain capacity in future
- Involve the patient to the maximum extent possible
- Consider (so far as reasonably ascertainable) past and present wishes and feelings of the patient, especially written wishes, and their relevant beliefs and values and other factors they would likely consider if able
- If practicable and appropriate, consult and take into account views of anyone named by the patient; this may include non-family members who may be carers
- Assess whether the act can be done in a less restrictive way.
- If issues concern life sustaining treatment, the determination should be in the patient's best interests, and not motivated by desire to bring about death

The Act provides a defence to what would otherwise be assault for the patient possessing capacity, in connection with the clinical care or treatment of the patient. It should be clarified that reasonable steps have been taken to establish that the patient indeed does lack capacity, and the action must be in the patient's best interests. It should be noted that a valid and applicable advance refusal take precedence.

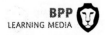

The determination of capacity should be within the remit of any clinician, however when there is sufficient doubt it may be reasonable to seek the help of a psychiatrist and the Trust legal team.

One example of an intervention is physical restraint of the patient. The latter is permissible only if necessary to prevent harm to the patient and this restraint should be proportionate to the likelihood and seriousness of harm. The restraint should be the most minimum that is required to achieve the desired outcome.

Lasting Power of Attorney (LPA) extends to welfare (including healthcare) matters, in addition to property and financial matters. The individual creating the contract (and for whom the LPA is created) is termed the donor, and the individual who is given LPA status is termed the donee. This contract must be in a prescribed form, and registered to include the certificate of capacity from an independent person. The LPA donor may place restrictions on powers, and may provide for replacement. The donee may not appoint a successor, nor delegate authority. The donee is empowered to make healthcare decisions only once the donor is incapacitated. An advance refusal outranks the LPA unless the LPA is created after the advance refusal, and the LPA is valid and applicable. Life sustaining treatment may be provided when there is conflict with the LPA, pending a Court decision. Therefore in the event of disagreement between the doctor and the donee with regard to treatment, there is an obligation on the doctor to pursue the case to Court if necessary. If there is evidence of a possible failure by a donee to act in the best interests of the donor, this should lead to a reference to the Public Guardian. In situations where LPAs are seen to be invalid, there is protection given to donees and third parties relying on these LPAs.

Advance refusals must be valid and applicable. They will not be valid if:

- They are subsequently withdrawn
- They are overridden by a subsequent applicable LPA
- The patient has acted in a way which is clearly inconsistent with the decision

- There were circumstances which existed which were not anticipated and these were likely to have affected the decision

Advance refusals may be overridden in order to provide treatment for a mental disorder of a patient detained formally under the Mental Health Act. It is for healthcare professionals to decide at first if the advance refusal is valid and applicable. If there are concerns, there is a duty of care to enquire to the Court of Protection. If the doctor reasonably believes that a valid and applicable advance refusal exists, there will be no liability if treatment is withheld. It is important however that if a doctor suspects that an advance refusal exists, reasonable efforts must be made, time permitting, to find out the detail; the doctor is permitted to act in the patient's best interests in an emergency.

Advance refusals only apply to refusals of treatment; patients may not make advance directives for specific treatments. It does not apply to life sustaining treatment unless it is stated in writing, and signed by or at the patient's direction and witnessed in writing.

Independent mental capacity advocates (IMCA) are instructed by an NHS body or local authority to represent and support an incapacitated patient before any decisions are made with regard to serious medical treatment, NHS arranged accommodation, a stay of 28 days or more in hospital, or a stay in a care home for 8 weeks or more. This applies where no-one appropriate exists for the NHS body or local authority to consult with. The role of the IMCA is to advise on the patient's best interests, wishes, and to obtain further information. The IMCA is entitled to meet the patient in private and view the medical records. Information or submissions from the IMCA must be taken into account when providing care. The IMCA may challenge a decision; this is referred to the Court of Protection.

It is important to remember that the issues of capacity relate not only to day-to-day clinical scenarios, but also to the issue of consent to research.

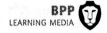

## *Seeking a patient's consent*

A good relationship between doctors and patients is built on trust. This is achieved by respecting the patients' autonomy, and their right to decide whether to undergo any medical intervention or not (even when their refusal may result in causing themselves harm or eventual death). This relates to the issues of capacity discussed above. When seeking their consent, patients must be provided with clear and sufficient information so that they can make an informed decision over their health care; effective communication is the key. The GMC suggests that the following points are addressed when seeking consent:

- Details of diagnosis and prognosis – and the likely prognosis if the condition is left untreated
- Uncertainties about the diagnosis including options for further investigation prior to treatment
- Options for treatment or management of the condition, including the option not to treat
- Purpose of the proposed investigation or treatment
- Details of the procedures or therapies involved, including:
  – Subsidiary treatment such as methods of pain relief
  – How the patient should prepare for the procedure
  – Details of what the patient might experience during or after the procedure including common and serious side effects
- Explanations of the likely benefits and the probabilities of success
- Discussion of any serious or frequently occurring risks, and of any lifestyle changes which may result from the treatment
- Advice about whether a proposed treatment is experimental
- How and when the patient's condition and any side effects will be monitored or re-assessed
- The name of the doctor who will have overall responsibility for the treatment
- Whether doctors undergoing training will be involved in delivering the treatment
- Reminder that the patient can change their minds about a decision at any point in time
- Reminder that the patient has the right to seek a second opinion
- Where applicable a discussion of the costs involved.

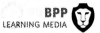

## Relevant questions – capacity

1.  How often is the issue of capacity relevant in your specialty?
2.  Which experts would you involve to help you decide whether your patient has capacity?
3.  A typical scenario may be discussed involving withdrawal of or lack of consent for an intervention.

## The non-commencement or withholding of medical treatment

Doctors have a responsibility to make the best interests of their patients their first concern. This is essential when considering any of the growing range of life-prolonging treatments which make it possible to extend the lives of patients who, through organ failure and life-threatening conditions, might otherwise die. The benefits of modern techniques such as cardiopulmonary resuscitation, renal dialysis, artificial ventilation, and artificial nutrition and hydration are considerable. However, any consideration for intervention has to be weighed against any perception that the natural end to life may be imminent (particularly with regard to chronic pathologies). The key word is often 'futility'. It is acceptable to withhold life-saving treatment if this same treatment is seen to be futile. However the definition of futility may be open to debate. Some would believe that in 'hopeless' cases with little or no hope of recovery, treatment may be withheld. Others would argue that the definition of 'hopeless' is open to debate, and treatment should only be withheld if the patient will definitely die despite the intervention. Often, reaching a satisfactory answer may mean addressing a number of difficult ethical and legal issues with the involvement of many different specialties and professions. The Trust legal team may have a role.

There may be some concerns in the public domain with regard to the possibility of over- or under-treatment towards the end of life. Some may feel that some doctors may make decisions about life-prolonging treatments without access to up to date clinical advice. It is also clear that the profession and patients want more guidance on what is considered ethically and legally permissible in this area. Patients and their families also want greater involvement

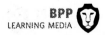

in making these decisions with better arrangements to support them when facing these distressing situations.

It should be stressed that when it has been agreed that a certain intervention should not be commenced, the patient should receive full care and attention up to the point of the futile intervention. It is a common misconception for example that when patients are labelled 'not for cardiopulmonary resuscitation', that they are not for treatment. This misunderstanding may lead to confusion, errors, poor treatment and complaints.

## End-of-life care

It may become obvious that the non-commencement or withholding of medical treatment may lead to the dying process. Alternatively active treatment may be withdrawn (de-escalated) when futility is obvious. It is paramount in these situations that the patient (who is often unconscious and therefore lacks capacity) and their significant others are fully involved and aware, and are left in no doubt about the situation. Clarity and effective communication are essential skills in this context. In my experience when communication here is clear, the relatives though devastated, fully understand the situation. When there seems to be lack of understanding every effort should be made to improve communication; this may involve the introduction of other personnel. A common misconception, unfortunately promoted even by some healthcare professionals, is that the decision to withdraw treatment rests with the family of a dying patient. It is important to highlight that this decision is a clinical one and that the duty of the doctor is to explain the issues of futility articulately to the family.

However if despite all efforts the relatives of the dying patient disagree with the treatment de-escalation plans, the matter may sadly have to be referred to the courts. It is fortunate that this scenario is rare.

Terminal care is defined as the care needed in the last few days of life. When this is embarked upon, high standards need to be adopted. The care may be best achieved when working collaboratively to facilitate a holistic approach:

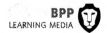

- Staff need to recognise that the care of the dying patient is an important and integral part of the care offered to patients within the trust
- Respect for patient autonomy, and informed decision-making in adults is promoted by honest and sensitive discussion with patients about care and treatment options. This includes helping those who wish to do so issue an advanced directive to inform future care at a time when they are no longer able to make decisions. Where this is not appropriate (eg confused or unconscious patients), discussion about care and treatment will occur with the family, taking into account previously known wishes and personal values of the patient
- Staff need to recognise the need for patients to have choice and control over where death occurs. This includes acknowledgement that some patients want their terminal care provided in the hospital setting. Other patients may wish to have their terminal care at home or in the hospice setting
- Visiting should be unrestricted for the terminal patient, and provision is made for relatives/carers to stay overnight with patients. Attention is paid to practical needs and concerns of patient, family, and friends
- Staff should aim to ensure that patients wishes are respected in relation to who should be present at the time of death, recognising that different cultures may have different needs
- Attention to pain relief, and other symptom control is recognised as a fundamental aspect of good terminal care
- Psychological, social, and spiritual support for patients and families is a vital component of care throughout the dying process and in bereavement
- All patients and staff should have access to the Trust's specialist Palliative Care Team if required
- All patients and relatives should have access to the Trust's multifaith Chaplaincy service and translation services if required
- Patients must be afforded dignity and privacy. This is given irrespective of age, disability, gender, race, sexual orientation, spiritual beliefs, etc
- Staff should receive support and education in order to offer an optimum service

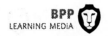

## *Relevant questions – treatment*

1. Have you recently been involved in the de-escalation or withholding of treatment for any of your patients? What was your role? Who did you involve? What was the outcome?
2. Are there circumstances in which withholding or withdrawing life-prolonging treatment would be unlawful?
3. With regard to the withholding of treatment, what are the responsibilities in the decision-making process of the patient, doctor, healthcare team, family members and other people who are close to the patient? What weight should be given to their views?

## Adverse incidents, medical error and complaints

The history, importance and philosophy of reporting adverse incidents and dealing with complaints have been dealt with in a previous chapter. Clearly there may be implications for legal action, and this will depend on the nature of the incident. The legal department of the Trust will normally take the lead in these cases, and will notify the relevant individuals. The responses in turn should be fed back to the Trust legal team, who then will be in a position to issue the Trust response.

It is also important to recognise that on discovery of an adverse incident, it may be relevant and prudent to inform the patient if there has been direct patient involvement; this should be done in a professional manner.

## *Relevant questions – legal cases*

1. Have you been involved in a legal case against the Trust? What was your role? How was the case resolved? Could the case have been handled better?
2. Can you describe how the Trust deals with legal cases?
3. Have you ever been charged with informing a patient about an adverse incident pertaining to his care?
4. A scenario may be discussed where a patient needs to be informed about an adverse incident pertaining to their care.

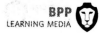

## Key points

You should be aware of the following principles:

- Assessing the capacity of a patient and seeking a patient's consent
- The non-commencement or withholding of medical treatment
- End-of-life care
- Openness in relation to adverse incidents, medical error and complaints

# Chapter 27

## Other key reports

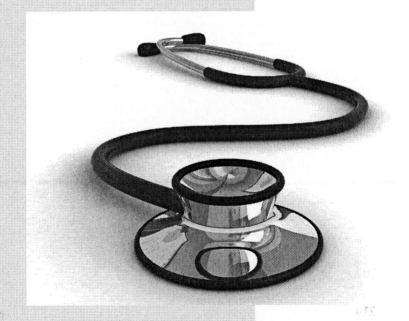

# Other key reports

Many important reports have been alluded to in previous chapters. The aim in identifying the additional reports below is to include those which had an impact on multiple and wide ranging topics.

## The Tooke Report: 'Aspiring to Excellence'

This was the final report of the independent inquiry into Modernising Medical Careers and was led by Professor Sir John Tooke. This was published in 2008.

The abstract of the report reads:

> *MMC sought to reform postgraduate medical education and training to speed the production of competent specialists. Reform comprised: a two year foundation programme; centralised selection into 'run- through' specialist training; the creation of fixed term specialist training appointments (FTSTAs); revisions to the non-consultant career grade. The Inquiry systematically analysed areas of concern arising from MMC: 1: Policy; 2: Professional engagement; 3: Workforce analysis; 4: Regulation; 5: Education and selection; 6: Training commissioning and management; 7: Service implications. The panel proposed corrective action to resolve issues in the eight domains listed below. The resulting Interim Report with its associated recommendations was published on 8 October 2007. Consultation on the Report revealed strong agreement. 87 per cent of the 1,440 respondents agreed or strongly agreed with the 45 recommendations.*
>
> (The Tooke Report, 2008)

The issues were as follows:

* The policy objective of postgraduate medical training was unclear. There was no consensus on the educational principles guiding postgraduate medical training. Moreover, there were no strong mechanisms for creating such consensus
* There was no consensus on the role of doctors at various career stages
* Weak DH policy development, implementation, and governance together with poor inter- and intra-Departmental

links adversely affected the planned reform of postgraduate training
- Medical workforce planning was hampered by lack of clarity regarding doctors' roles and did not align with other aspects of health policy. There was no structured policy regarding the potential massive increase in trainee numbers. Planning capacity was limited and training commissioning budgets were vulnerable in England, as they were held at SHA level
- The medical profession's effective involvement in training policy-making had been weak
- The management of postgraduate training was hampered by unclear principles, a weak contractual base, a lack of cohesion, a fragmented structure, and in England, deficient relationships with academia and service
- The regulation of the continuum of medical education involved two bodies: GMC and PMETB, creating diseconomies in terms of both finance and expertise
- The structure of postgraduate training proposed by MMC was unlikely to encourage or reward striving for excellence, offer appropriate flexibility to trainees, facilitate future work-force design, or meet the needs of particular groups (eg those with academic aspirations, or those pursuing a non-consultant career grade experience). It risked creating another 'lost tribe' at FTSTA level

Corrective action:

- There should be clear shared principles for postgraduate medical training that emphasise flexibility and an aspiration to excellence
- Consensus on the role of doctors needed to be reached quickly, and the service contribution of trainees better acknowledged
- DH policy development, implementation and governance should be strengthened. DH should appoint a lead for medical education, and strengthen collaboration
- Workforce policy objectives should be integrated with training and service objectives. Medical workforce advisory machinery should be revised and enhanced. SHA workforce planning and commissioning should be subject to external scrutiny.

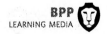

Policies with respect to the current bulge in trainees and international medical graduates should be urgently resolved

- The profession should develop a mechanism for providing coherent advice on matters affecting the entire profession.
- The accountability structure for postgraduate training and funding flows should be reviewed. Revised management structures should conform to agreed principles but reflect local circumstances. In England 'Graduate Schools' should be trialled where supported locally
- PMETB should be merged within GMC to facilitate economies of scale, a common approach, linkage of accreditation with registration and the sharing of quality enhancement expertise
- The structure of postgraduate training should be modified to provide a broad based platform for subsequent higher specialist training, increased flexibility, the valuing of experience and the promotion of excellence

Conclusion:

*To deal with many of the deficiencies identified and to ensure the necessary concerted action, the creation of a new body, NHS: Medical Education England (NHS:MEE) is proposed. NHS:MEE will relate to the revised medical workforce advisory machinery and act as the professional interface between policy development and implementation on matters relating to PGMET. It will promote national cohesion in England as well as working with equivalent bodies in the Devolved Administrations to facilitate UK wide collaboration. The Inquiry has charted a way forward and received a strong professional mandate. The recommendations and the aspiration to excellence they represent must not be lost in translation. NHS:MEE will help assure their implementation.*

(The Tooke Report, 2008)

The recommendations and conclusion of the report were accepted in principle, and plans for the merger of GMC and PMETB are already afoot, as described in a previous chapter.

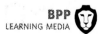

## *Ara Darzi's Reports*

In December 2006, NHS London (the Strategic Health Authority for London) asked Professor Lord Darzi to develop a strategy to meet Londoners' health needs over the following 5 to 10 years. Lord Darzi identified reasons why the time was right for a co-ordinated programme of change across London. The main driver for this report was the perception that inequalities were rife in London, and that Londoners were not satisfied with health care. Lord Darzi (Sir Ara Darzi as he was then) set out a vision for change, and in July 2007 produced a report titled *A Framework for Action*. The subject matter focused on:

- The plans to tackle the predicted growth in population, particularly in the aged
- Services focused on individual needs and choices
- The philosophy of 'localise where possible, centralise where necessary', with regard to the provision of primary to tertiary health care
- Truly integrated care and partnership working, maximising the contribution of the entire workforce
- The philosophy that prevention is better than cure
- A focus on health inequalities and diversity
- A vision on models of health care, ranging from rehabilitation at home, through polyclinics to acute academic tertiary centres

In 2008, Lord Darzi published another repor, *High Quality Care for All*. This was the final report of the NHS Next Stage Review, co-produced with the NHS during a year-long process involving more than 2,000 clinicians and 60,000 NHS staff, patients, stakeholders and members of the public. High quality care has always been a guiding principle for NHS staff. However, in the last 10 years, much of the focus has been on building capacity. Following this significant investment in resources, the time was considered right to align the system to support the delivery of high quality care by frontline staff. Lord Darzi defines quality of care as clinically effective, personal and safe. This means protecting patient safety by eradicating healthcare acquired infections and avoidable accidents. It is about effectiveness of care, from the clinical procedure the patient receives to their quality of life after treatment. It is also about the patient's entire experience of the NHS and ensuring

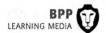

they are treated with compassion, dignity and respect in a clean, safe and well-managed environment. It is likely that many of the philosophies of Lord Darzi will apply to the evolution of health care in England within and outside London.

## The Kennedy Report

From the late 1980s onwards, concerns about the performance of the Bristol Paediatric Cardiothoracic Unit were increasingly expressed in a variety of contexts. Some of these concerns were from healthcare professionals working in the Unit, while others were expressed by individuals in a variety of contexts outside the Unit. Rumours were common, and some appeared in the form of unattributed reports in the media. An operation performed on Joshua Loveday on 12 January 1995 proved to be the catalyst for further action. Joshua died on the operating table, and an external review was instituted. Complaints were subsequently made to the GMC concerning the conduct of two cardiac surgeons and of the Chief Executive of the Trust. They were found guilty in 1998 of serious professional misconduct. A group of parents of children who had undergone cardiac surgery at the BRI organised themselves to provide mutual support. In June 1996 the group first called for a Public Inquiry into the PCS services at the BRI.

The Kennedy report was published by the Bristol Royal Infirmary Inquiry in July 2001. The remit was:

- To inquire into the management of the care of children receiving complex cardiac surgical services at the Bristol Royal Infirmary between 1984 and 1995 and relevant related issues
- To make findings as to the adequacy of the services provided
- To establish what action was taken both within and outside the hospital to deal with concerns raised about the surgery
- To identify any failure to take appropriate action promptly
- To reach conclusions from these events
- To make recommendations which could help to secure high quality care across the NHS

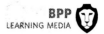

The Public Inquiry was conducted between October 1998 and July 2001. The panel was chaired by Professor Ian Kennedy.

There were many recommendations. The significant ones included:

- The clinical process: patients should receive copies of any letters which are written about them; there was also the suggestion that patients should be offered the facility to make tape recordings of consultations
- Informed consent: consent should be obtained for all examinations or procedures that involve any touching or physical contact with the patient
- Working with other professional groups: the need for good clinical governance was demonstrated
- Professional competence: the report revealed many failures of communication with patients and colleagues affecting all professional groups, and highlighted the need for instruction in communication skills for all healthcare professionals. The report, in emphasising the need for team work, recommended formal assessment of all aspects of competence including non-clinical elements of care, and placed continuing professional development (CPD) at the very centre of systems for assuring competence. Recommendations were also made for compulsory periodic appraisal for all health care professionals
- Local teams and professional barriers: the report highlighted the increasing need for healthcare professionals to work in multidisciplinary teams, and demonstrated many failures that arose from continued barriers between professional groups. Amongst the measures recommended by the report were the value of shared learning across professional boundaries, clinical audit, reflective practice, and leadership
- Monitoring standards and performance: multidisciplinary clinical audit was identified as a core vehicle for monitoring local performance
- Adverse events and a 'no blame culture': recommendations were made that individual employees should be immune from disciplinary action when reporting adverse events. Please note though that, as mentioned in relevant chapters, it has been recognised that reporting adverse events should carry 'appropriate blame' to ensure that appropriate actions are taken following incidents

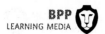

- The external climate of the NHS: the report also served to highlight contributions to the Bristol tragedy made by under-funding and the concentration by governments on containing costs
- Doctors and management: doctors engaged in management should be given sufficient time within their contracted hours
- to carry out those duties and they should receive specific training for the work

It is clear that this report has relevance to many themes discussed elsewhere in this book.

## The Francis Report

Robert Francis QC published his inquiry report into the Mid-Staffordshire NHS Foundation Trust, following concerns about standards of care at the Trust, and an investigation and report published by the Healthcare Commission in March 2009. Robert Francis heard evidence from patients, their relatives and staff to inform his report. The Department of Health and the Trust Board accepted the recommendations of the Inquiry in full.

The reports were published to support all NHS organisations to learn from and respond to the recommendations of the report, and prevent such serious failures occurring again. These reports were:

### Review of Early Warning Systems in the NHS

This describes the systems and processes, and values and behaviours which make up a system for the early detection and prevention of serious failures in the NHS. It emphasises that everyone has a role to play – from doctors and nurses, to commissioners in PCTs, system managers in SHAs and DH, and the regulators – in safeguarding quality of care to patients

### Assuring the quality of senior NHS managers

This report of a working group sets out recommendations to further raise the standards of senior NHS managers. The report recognises that while the overwhelming majority of NHS managers

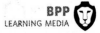

meet high professional standards every day, a very small number occasionally demonstrate performance or conduct that lets down the patients they serve as well as their staff and organisations. The group's recommendations include replacing the Code of Conduct for NHS managers with a new statement of professional ethics and consultation on a system of professional accreditation for senior NHS managers.

## The Healthy NHS Board

The document sets out the guiding principles that will allow NHS board members to understand the collective role of the board, governance within the wider NHS, approaches that are most likely to improve board effectiveness, and the contribution expected of individual board members.

Responding to some of the specific recommendations in the report, the Secretary of State accepted Robert Francis's recommendation to consider asking Monitor to de-authorise *Mid-Staffordshire NHS Foundation Trust.*

The Inquiry raised questions over the role of external organisations. Recommendation 16 of the report recommends a further Independent Inquiry of the commissioning, supervisory and regulatory bodies.

The report highlights the consequences of poor board performance on patient care and recommendation 9 makes clear the need for a regulatory and accreditation scheme for senior NHS managers that mirrors those in place for clinicians and nursing staff. One of the proposals contained in assuring the quality of NHS senior managers is to consult on a new system of accreditation for managers that aims to provide stronger assurance of the quality of senior managers in the NHS.

In response to the complicated issue of Hospital Standardised Mortality Ratios (HSMRs) Professor Sir Bruce Keogh, NHS Medical Director, established a working group and develop a single HSMR methodology for the NHS, which was raised in the Inquiry report.

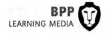

## Specific recommendations:

1. The Trust must make its first priority the delivery of a high-class standard of care to all its patients by putting their needs first. It should not provide a service where it cannot achieve this standard.

2. The Secretary of State for Health should consider whether he ought to request that Monitor – under the provisions of the Health Act 2009 – exercise its power of de-authorisation over the Mid Staffordshire NHS Foundation Trust. In the event of his deciding that continuation of foundation trust status is appropriate, the Secretary of State should keep that decision under review.

3. The Trust, together with the Primary Care Trust, should promote the development of links with other NHS trusts and foundation trusts to enhance its ability to deliver up-to-date and high-class standards of service provision and professional leadership.

4. The Trust, in conjunction with the Royal Colleges, the Deanery and the nursing school at Staffordshire University, should review its training programmes for all staff to ensure that high-quality professional training and development is provided at all levels to and that high-quality service is recognised and valued.

5. The Board should institute a programme of improving the arrangements for audit in all clinical departments and make participation in audit processes in accordance with contemporary standards of practice a requirement for all relevant staff. The Board should review audit processes and outcomes on a regular basis.

6. The Board should review the Trust's arrangements for the management of complaints and incident reporting in the light of the findings of this report and ensure that it:
    a. Provides responses and resolutions to complaints which satisfy complainants;
    b. Ensures that staff are engaged from the investigation of a complaint or an incident to the implementation of any lessons to be learned all part of the recommendation;
    c. Minimises the risk of deficiencies exposed by the problems recurring; and makes available full information on the matters reported, and the action to resolve deficiencies, to the Board, the governors and the public.

7.    Trust policies, procedures and practice regarding professional oversight and discipline should be reviewed in the light of the principles described in this report.

8.    The Board should give priority to ensuring that any member of staff who raises an honestly held concern about the standard or safety of the provision of services to patients is supported and protected from any adverse consequences, and should foster a culture of openness and insight.

9.    In the light of the findings of this report, the Secretary of State and Monitor should review the arrangements for the training, appointment, support and accountability of executive and non-executive directors of NHS trusts and NHS foundation trusts, with a view to creating and enforcing uniform professional standards for such posts by means of standards formulated and overseen by an independent body given powers of disciplinary sanction.

10.   The Board should review the management/leadership of nursing staff to ensure that the principles described are complied with.

11.   The Board should review the management structure to ensure that clinical staff are fully represented at all levels of the Trust and that they are aware of concerns raised by clinicians on matters relating to the standard and safety of the service provided to patients.

12.   The Trust should review its record-keeping procedures in consultation with the clinical and nursing staff and regularly audit the standards of performance.

13.   All wards admitting elderly, acutely ill patients in significant numbers should have multidisciplinary meetings, with consultant medical input, on a weekly basis. The level of specialist elderly care medical input should also be reviewed, and all nursing staff (including healthcare assistants) should have training in the diagnosis and management of acute confusion.

14.   The Trust should ensure that its nurses work to a published set of principles, focusing on safe patient care.

15.   In view of the uncertainties surrounding the use of comparative mortality statistics in assessing hospital performance and the understanding of the term 'excess' deaths, an independent working group should be set up by the Department of Health to examine and report on the methodologies in use.

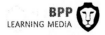

It should make recommendations as to how such mortality statistics should be collected, analysed and published, both to promote public confidence and understanding of the process, and to assist hospitals in using statistics as a prompt to examine areas of patient care.

16. The Department of Health should consider instigating an independent examination of the operation of commissioning, supervisory and regulatory bodies in relation to their monitoring role at Stafford hospital with the objective of learning lessons about how failing hospitals are identified.

17. The Trust and the Primary Care Trust should consider steps to enhance the rebuilding of public confidence in the Trust.

18. All NHS Trusts and Foundation Trusts responsible for the provision of hospital services should review their standards, governance and performance in the light of this report.

All acute trusts are now examining ways to properly implement the findings of the report. It is important to build an awareness of the Francis Report with regard to the running of your department and the implementation of any cost-saving projects.

## The White Paper 'Equity and Excellence: Liberating the NHS'

After the election in May 2010, one of the first acts of the new Conservative-Liberal Democrat coalition government was, with immediate effect, to reduce the emergency care target threshold from 98 per cent to 95 per cent; waiting time targets to see a GP were removed altogether. All other targets are in a state of flux, and the exact nature of the final recommendations are unclear at the time of writing. The following is a summary of what is proposed.

There are some significant cost reduction targets for the NHS; these are currently focussed around reducing overhead and management costs, and the hope is that in the long term there will be significant cost reduction by improved efficiency, as a consequence of the changes outlined below.

The White Paper was presumably constructed to reinforce the philosophy of the new government, and was published on 12 July 2010, setting out the Government's strategy for the NHS.

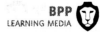

The White Paper sought views on the policies included, in particular on the following:

- Commissioning for Patients
- Freeing Providers and Economic Regulation
- Local Democratic Legitimacy in Health
- The Review of Arm's-Length Bodies
- The NHS Outcomes Framework

The overall purpose was to:

- Put patients and the public first
- Focus on improvement in quality and healthcare outcomes
- Promote autonomy, accountability and democratic legitimacy (see below)
- Cut bureaucracy and increase efficiency

Introducing an NHS Outcomes Framework will (not surprisingly) attempt to achieve improved outcomes. It will also enable the Secretary of State to hold the NHS Commissioning Board to account. This will mean that the NHS Commissioning Board, GP consortia, patients and the public will all have better information about the quality of services delivered by individual providers.

The White Paper will attempt to increase autonomy within the NHS, enable decisions to be made at the most appropriate level and empower providers and clinicians within them. Providers will be given the freedom to respond to patient needs and preferences. Moving commissioning functions to GP consortia will mean that there is greater alignment between clinical decision making and the financial consequences of these decisions. Increased autonomy will be accompanied by greater accountability, to patients, the public and others within the health system.

Cutting bureaucracy and increasing efficiency is predominantly about making better use of available resources. Within the arm's length body sector, there are currently 18 organisations, whose functions often overlap. To both simplify the system and to save money, this was thought to need to be rationalisation. The same also applies to other areas, such as central programmes.

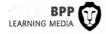

Unnecessary bureaucracy associated with medical research and data returns will also be removed.

Abolition of PCTs and SHAs were planned for 2013, with commissioning at local level transferring to GP clusters (consortia) and overseen by a National Commissioning Board. At the time of writing, SHAs may perhaps be replaced by regional arms of the Commissioning Board. The role of the NHS Commissioning Board includes:

- Allocation of resources to GP consortia
- Overseeing the workings of GP consortia
- Liaising with Local Authority
- Direct commissioning for specialised services eg primary care, maternity
- Providing a less 'hands on' approach than SHA ie gives more independence to GP consortia
- Being more independent than SHAs

GP consortia should remove some duplication of functions previously administered by PCTs and practice-based commissioners. Commissioning by GP consortia will most probably employ similar models to those used by PCTs. Providers will be within the domains of primary and secondary care as before.

The Care Quality Commission (CQC) will oversee standards in healthcare provision (primary and secondary care) and commissioning as before. 'Monitor' (the Independent Regulator of NHS Foundation Trusts) will take on an expanded role. It will, in addition to its present remit of assessing trusts applying for Foundation status and overseeing standards in Foundation Trusts, also concentrate on patient welfare. Emphasis is to be placed on all trusts achieving foundation trust status. Patients' choice will be strengthened by rewarding responsive providers and the creation of a robust information strategy.

**Key points**

You should be aware of the following reports and papers:

- The Tooke Report *Aspiring to Excellence* (dealing with training, education and roles)
- The Darzi Report (dealing with growth in population; needs and choices; integrated care and partnership working; health inequalities and diversity; and models of health care)
- The Kennedy Report (dealing with patient inclusion; informed consent; good clinical governance; professional competence; local teams and professional barriers; monitoring standards and performance; adverse events and a 'no blame culture'; the external climate of the NHS; and doctors and management)
- The Francis Report (dealing with early warning systems, quality of management, quality of Trust Boards)
- The White Paper *Equity and Excellence: Liberating the NHS* (dealing with commissioning modernisation)

# Section 6

## Ending the interview

# Ending the interview

At the end of the interview you will almost certainly be asked, 'Do you wish to ask the panel anything?' It is vital that you do not undo all the good work that you have done. What you say at the end of your interview before you depart will leave a lasting impression on the members of the panel.

It may be appropriate to use questions as a vehicle to:

- Qualify or amplify a previous point
- Correct an earlier answer
- Clarify that you have no questions, as key personnel have dealt with your queries during your formal visit

If you are appointed, there will be plenty of scope to have discussions with Medical Personnel in the time leading up to commencement of the job. It is therefore not appropriate to mention salaries or annual leave. It is perfectly acceptable to say 'I don't have any questions'.

When making your exit, you should make a point of acknowledging as many of the panel as possible. This may be manifested as a small nod and a 'thank you' addressed to the panel as a whole. When leaving, ensure you remember which door to exit from, if there is more than one. Walking into a broom cupboard will not leave the right kind of lasting impression.

 **Key points**
- Choose your words carefully when asked if you have any questions
- It is perfectly acceptable to say 'I don't have any questions'
- Ending the interview: try to leave a lasting impression which is professional and courteous

# Appendix

## References
## Useful websites

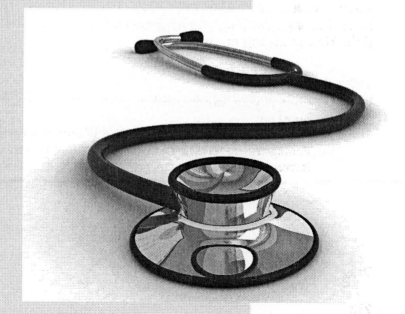

# References

## *Adverse healthcare events and risk*

- Department of Health. *An organisation with a memory* (June 2007) London: HMSO [Online] Available at www. dh.gov.uk/en/Publicationsandstatistics/Publications/ PublicationsPolicyAndGuidance/DH_4065083 [Accessed 17/11/11].
- Department of Health. *Building a safer NHS for patients: Implementing an organisation with a memory* (April 2002) London: HMSO [Online] Available at www.dh.gov. uk/en/Publicationsandstatistics/Publications/ PublicationsPolicyAndGuidance/DH_4097460 [Accessed 17/11/11].

## *The internal market*

Department of Health. White Paper: *Working for Patients.* HAA 0165 0145 (Jan 1989); London: HMSO (Cm 555).

## *The NHS Plan, precursors and consequences*

- Department of Health. *The Health of the Nation. A strategy for health in England* (July 1992) London HMSO (Cm1986).
- Department of Health. *The new NHS – Modern, Dependable* (1997) London: HMSO (Cm 3807).
- Department of Health. *The NHS Plan. A plan for investment, a plan for reform* (July 2000) London: HMSO [Online] Available at www.dh.gov.uk/en/Publicationsandstatistics/Publications/ PublicationsPolicyAndGuidance/DH_4002960 [Accessed 17/11/11].
- Department of Health. *Securing our future health: taking a long-term view – the Wanless report* (April 2002) London: HMSO [Online] Available at www.dh.gov.uk/en/Publicationsandstatistics/ Publications/PublicationsPolicyAndGuidance/DH_4009293 [Accessed 17/11/11].

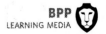

## Protecting electronic patient information

BMA/NHS Connecting for Health. *Joint Guidance on Protecting Electronic Patient Information* [Online] Available at www.connectingforhealth.nhs.uk/systemsandservices/infogov/links/jointguidance.pdf [Accessed 17/11/11].

## Reports

### The Griffiths Report

Griffiths R et al. *NHS Management Inquiry*. Letter dated 6 October 1983 to the Secretary of State, Norman Fowler. [Online] Available at www.sochealth.co.uk/history/griffiths.htm [Accessed 17/11/10].

### The Ara Darzi Report

Darzi A. *A framework for action*. London:NHS London [Online] Available at www.nhshistory.net/darzilondon.pdf [Accessed 17/11/11].

### The Kennedy Report

Kennedy I. *The Bristol Inquiry* [Online] Available at www.bristol-inquiry.org.uk [Accessed 17/11/11].

### The Francis Report

Francis R. *Robert Francis Inquiry report into Mid-Staffordshire NHS Foundation Trust* (February 2010) [Online] Available at www.dh.gov.uk/en/Publicationsandstatistics/Publications/PublicationsPolicyAndGuidance/DH_113018 [Accesssed 17/11/11].

### The Tooke Report

Tooke J. *Aspring to excellence: final report into the independent inquiry into Modernising Medical Careers* [Online] Available at www.mmcinquiry.org.uk/MMC_FINAL_REPORT_REVD_4jan.pdf [Accessed 17/11/11].

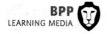

## The Royal Liverpool Children's Inquiry

[Online] Available at www.rlcinquiry.org.uk [Accessed 17/11/11].

## *Other references*

Department of Health. *Best Research for Best Health: A new national health research strategy* (February 2007) [Online] Available at www.dh.gov.uk/en/Publicationsandstatistics/Publications/PublicationsPolicyAndGuidance/Browsable/DH_4127225 [Accessed 17/11/11].

Department of Health. *The White Paper, Equity and excellence: Liberating the NHS* (July 2010) [Online] Available at www.dh.gov.uk/en/Publicationsandstatistics/Publications/PublicationsPolicyAndGuidance/DH_117353 [Accessed 17/11/11].

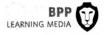

# Useful websites

## *Care Quality Commission*
www.cqc.org.uk

## *Clinical audit*
www.hqip.org.uk/what-is-clinical-audit

## *Clinical governance*
www.webarchive.nationalarchives.gov.uk/+/www.dh.gov.uk/en/
Publichealth/Patientsafety/Clinicalgovernance/index.htm

## *HaN*
www.healthcareworkforce.nhs.uk/hospitalatnight.html

## *Healthcare resource groups and 'Payment by Results' (the Casemix Service)*
www.ic.nhs.uk/casemix

## *The Human Tissue Act (2004)*
www.hta.gov.uk/legislationpoliciesandcodesofpractice/legislation/
humantissueact.cfm

## *Mental Capacity Act (2005)*
www.dh.gov.uk/en/SocialCare/Deliveringsocialcare/
MentalCapacity/MentalCapacityAct2005/index.htm

## *The MLCF*
www.institute.nhs.uk/assessment_tool/general/medical_
leadership_competency_framework_-_homepage.html

## *MMC*
www.mmc.nhs.uk

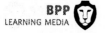

## *National Service frameworks and strategies*
www.nhs.uk/nhsengland/NSF/pages/Nationalserviceframeworks.aspx

## *NHS Direct*
www.nhsdirect.nhs.uk/

## *NICE*
www.nice.org.uk

## *Patient Advocacy and Liaison Service (PALS)*
www.pals.nhs.uk

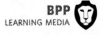

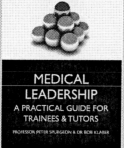
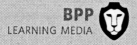

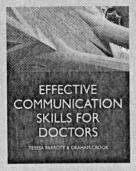
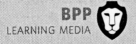

# More titles in the Progressing your Medical Career Series

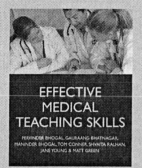

## EFFECTIVE MEDICAL TEACHING SKILLS

PERVINDER BHOGAL, GAURAANG BHATNAGAR, MANINDER BHOGAL, TOM CONNER, SHVAITA RALHAN, JANE YOUNG & MATT GREEN

*We can all remember a teacher that inspired us, encouraged us and helped us to excel. But what is it that makes a good teacher and are these skills that can be learned and improved?*

As doctors and healthcare professionals we are all expected to teach, to a greater or lesser degree, and this carries a great deal of responsibility. We are helping to develop the next generation and it is essential to pass on the knowledge that we have gained during our experience to date.

This book aims to cover the fundamentals of medical education. It has been designed to be a guide for the budding teacher with practical advice, hints, tips and essential points of reflection designed to encourage the reader to think about what they are doing at each step.

£19.99

October 2011

Paperback

978-1-445379-55-5

By taking the time to read through this book and completing the exercises contained within it you should:

- Understand the needs of the learner
- Understand the skills required to be an effective teacher
- Understand the various different teaching scenarios, from lectures to problem based teaching, and how to use them effectively
- Understand the importance and sources of feedback
- Be aware of assessment techniques, appraisal and revalidation

This book aims to provide you with a foundation in medical education upon which you can build the skills and attributes to become a competent and skilled teacher.

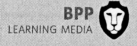

**BPP** LEARNING MEDIA

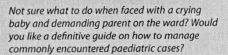
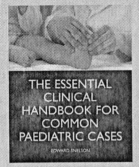
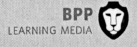

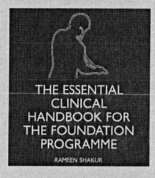
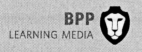

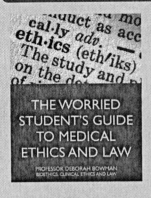
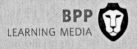

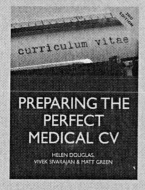
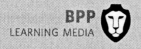

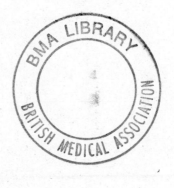